Antiphospholipid Syndrome Handbook

Maria Laura Bertolaccini,
Oier Ateka-Barrutia, and
Munther A. Khamashta

Antiphospholipid Syndrome Handbook

Springer

Maria Laura Bertolaccini, MD, PhD
Lupus Research Unit
The Rayne Institute
King's College London School of Medicine
St. Thomas' Hospital
London
UK

Oier Ateka-Barrutia, MD
Hospital de Navarra
Pamplona
Spain

Munther A. Khamashta, MD, FRCP, PhD
Lupus Unit
King's College London School of Medicine
St Thomas' Hospital
London
UK

ISBN 978-1-84628-522-6 e-ISBN 978-1-84628-735-0
DOI 10.1007/978-1-84628-735-0
Springer London Dordrecht Heidelberg New York

British Library Cataloguing in Publication Data
A catalogue record for this book is available from the British Library

Library of Congress Control Number: 2009932752

Printed on acid-free paper

Springer is part of Springer Science+Business Media (www.springer.com)

Foreword

The antiphospholipid syndrome (Hughes syndrome) is now over a quarter of a century old. Although most of the major clinical features were described in the original papers between 1983 and 1985, the ensuing 25 years have seen a filling out of the clinical detail and recognition that the syndrome is of major medical importance.

More significantly, much has been learnt of the prevalence and epidemiology of the syndrome as well as the biology of the thrombotic process so central to the condition. Sadly, all that lags behind is treatment, the choice of drugs still very limited.

The syndrome now embraces all disciplines. It is now regarded as the commonest treatable cause of recurrent pregnancy loss, and has changed the face of obstetrics. It has become a major chapter in the field of neurology, being an important cause of stroke, migraine, seizures, and memory loss. In cardiology, it is at last becoming recognized as an important cause of young heart attacks, as well as providing leads in the study of accelerated atheroma.

And so the list goes on – idiopathic bone fracture, abdominal angina, renal vascular hypertension, leg ulcers…

This book, produced by clinical leaders in the field, brings together the many strands of another "great mimic".

Graham R.V. Hughes

Contents

Chapter 1
History

The antiphospholipid syndrome (APS), first described in 1983 by Dr. Graham Hughes and his team at the Hammersmith Hospital, included recurrent arterial and venous thromboses, fetal losses, and thrombocytopenia in the presence of autoantibodies, the so-called antiphospholipid antibodies (aPL). Although a wide variety of clinical manifestations have been added over the last 5 years, these major features have stood the test of time. Many patients with APS have clinical and laboratory features common to other autoimmune diseases, particularly systemic lupus erythematosus (SLE). Such patients are defined as having secondary APS to distinguish them from patients with features of APS alone (primary APS-PAPS). There appears to be very few differences, if any, between the clinical complications associated with the primary and the secondary form of the syndrome, and the rates of arterial or venous thrombosis or fetal loss do not appear to be different. Distinguishing between PAPS and APS due to SLE can sometimes be difficult since many features, such as thrombocytopenia, anemia, renal, and central nervous system involvement, can be seen in both the conditions.

Historical description of aPL is summarized in Table 1.1.

M.L. Bertolaccini et al., *Antiphospholipid Syndrome Handbook*,
DOI 10.1007/978-1-84628-735-0_1,

TABLE 1.1. Historical description of antiphospholipid antibodies (aPL).

1906	Wasserman reaction (reagin)
1941	Reagin binds cardiolipin
1952	False-positive test for syphilis
1952	Lupus anticoagulant (LA)
1960s	LA: association with thrombosis
1970s	LA: association with fetal loss
1983	Anticardiolipin antibody (aCL)
1980s	Detailed description of anti phospholipid syndrome (APS)
1990	Phospholipid binding proteins (β2GPI)
1990s	Animal models for APS
1999	Classification criteria for definite APS
2006	Classification criteria updated

References

Harris EN, Gharavi AE, Boey ML, Patel BM, Mackworth-Young CG, Loizou S et al (1983) Anticardiolipin antibodies: detection by radioimmunoassay and association with thrombosis in systemic lupus erythematosus. Lancet 2(8361):1211–1214

Hughes GRV (1983) Thrombosis, abortion, cerebral disease, and the lupus anticoagulant. Br Med J 287(6399):1088–1089

Chapter 2
Epidemiology

The prevalence of antiphospholipid antibodies (aPL) in otherwise healthy populations is less than 1%. Many autoantibodies become more prevalent with increasing age and aPL is no exception. aPL has been reported in 10–20% of the healthy elderly population.

In autoimmune diseases, especially SLE, however, the prevalence is much higher. The Euro-Lupus study found a prevalence of 24% for IgG anticardiolipin antibody (aCL), 13% for IgM aCL, and 15% for lupus anticoagulant (LA), respectively, in a cohort of 1,000 patients with SLE. A recent study showed that the prevalence of antiphospholipid syndrome (APS) increases from 10 to 23% after 15–18 years in a large cohort of SLE patients.

In patients with unselected venous thromboembolism, the prevalence of aCL varies from 3 to 17% and 3 to 14% for the LA. Around 18% of young patients with stroke (<40 years old) are positive for aPL, whereas the APASS study found that 9.7% of first stroke patients had a positive aCL. In myocardial infarction, the prevalence of aCL is between 5 and 15%. Multiple cross-sectional studies have reported an association of aCL and/or LA with recurrent fetal loss (ranging from 10 to 20%).

There are numerous traps for the unwary and many other conditions can be associated with aPL but are not necessarily associated with thrombosis. Thus aPL may occur in infections such as HIV and malignancy and may also follow exposure to

M.L. Bertolaccini et al., *Antiphospholipid Syndrome Handbook*,
DOI 10.1007/978-1-84628-735-0_2,

certain drugs. aPL in these circumstances are not necessarily pathogenic, and these conditions should therefore be considered in any differential diagnosis of APS. The significance of these autoantibodies remains unclear and could be related to the increasing prevalence of associated conditions in the elderly such as malignancy and drug treatment.

References

Cervera R, Khamashta MA, Font J, Sebastiani GD, Gil A, Lavilla P et al (2003) Morbidity and mortality in systemic lupus erythematosus during a 10-year period: a comparison of early and late manifestations in a cohort of 1, 000 patients. Medicine (Baltimore) 82(5):299–308

Cervera R, Piette JC, Font J, Khamashta MA, Shoenfeld Y, Camps MT et al (2002) Antiphospholipid syndrome: clinical and immunologic manifestations and patterns of disease expression in a cohort of 1, 000 patients. Arthritis Rheum 46(4):1019–1027

Chapter 3
Antiphospholipid Antibodies

Phospholipids are a class of polar lipid components of cell membranes. They play an important role in the clotting cascade. Their presence is critical at several points in the extrinsic, intrinsic, and common pathways of coagulation. Phospholipids are required for the activation of factors IX (intrinsic pathway) and for the activation of factor X, and the conversion from prothrombin to thrombin (common pathway) (Fig. 3.1).

Although direct evidence for a pathophysiologic role of antiphospholipid antibodies (aPLs) is lacking, it is hypothesized that autoantibodies to phospholipid-binding proteins contribute directly to a thrombotic diathesis by interfering with hemostatic reactions that occur on anionic phospholipid membranes in vivo.

aPLs are a family of immunoglobulins of IgG, IgM, IgA, or a combination of these isotypes, which were initially thought to recognize anionic phospholipids. Over the years, this concept has changed and different specificities have been described for aPL (Table 3.1).

3.1 Anticardiolipin Antibodies

Cardiolipin is an anionic phospholipid, historically important as an antigen for testing reagin in syphilis serology. Currently, it is a part of the antigenic composition used in the VDRL tests along with lecithin and cholesterol.

M.L. Bertolaccini et al., *Antiphospholipid Syndrome Handbook*,
DOI 10.1007/978-1-84628-735-0_3,

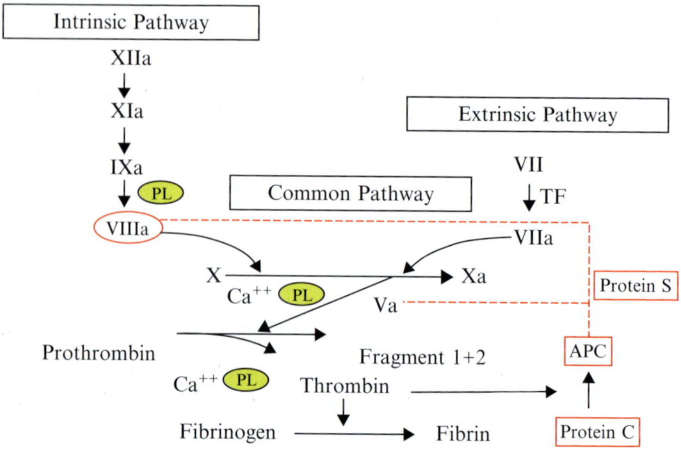

FIG. 3.1. Phospholipid involvement in the coagulation cascade.

TABLE 3.1. Different aPL specificities.

Antiphospholipid antibodies
Reagin
Antibodies to anionic phospholipids
Cardiolipin
Phosphatidylserine
Phosphatidic acid
Phosphatidylinositol
Antibodies to neutral phospholipids
Phosphatidylcholine
Antibodies to zwitteronic phospholipids
Phosphatidylethanolamine
Antibodies to phospholipid binding proteins
β2GPI
Prothrombin
Annexin V
Protein C
Protein S
Low molecular weight kininogens
High molecular weight kininogens

In 1983, Harris et al. developed a solid-phase radioimmunoassay to detect aCL using cardiolipin as antigen. This assay proved to be more sensitive than the classical VDRL in detecting aPL. However, in addition to detecting aCL, this assay also detects antibodies to serum or plasma proteins that bind to cardiolipin coated to the plate, in particular, antibodies to β2-glycoprotein I (anti-β2GPI).

3.2 Lupus Anticoagulant

LA is a functional measurement of the capacity of heterogeneous aPL that interfere with phospholipid-dependent stages of blood coagulation in vitro and inhibit both the intrinsic and common pathways of coagulation. Paradoxically, LAs are associated with a thrombotic tendency rather than bleeding, generally associated with coagulation inhibitors.

Testing for LA is a tedious task. Their heterogeneous nature makes it necessary to perform more than one coagulation test to reach the diagnosis according to the classification criteria. A number of features need to be demonstrated: (1) prolongation of a phospholipid-dependent clotting time; (2) evidence of inhibition shown by mixing studies; (3) evidence of phospholipid dependence; and (4) exclusion of specific inhibition of any one coagulation factor. In principle, the laboratory tests to detect the LA should use a sensitive screening test followed by a specific confirmation test. An algorithm for the detection of LA is shown in Fig. 3.2.

3.3 Other aPL

3.3.1 Anti-β2GPI Antibodies

In 1990, three independent groups identified β2GPI as the plasma cofactor required for aCL binding to cardiolipin. β2GPI is a normal plasma glycoprotein, a single-chain 50 kD polypeptide. Its function is unclear, although it may function as a natural anticoagulant. β2GPI antibodies are more specific than aCL in

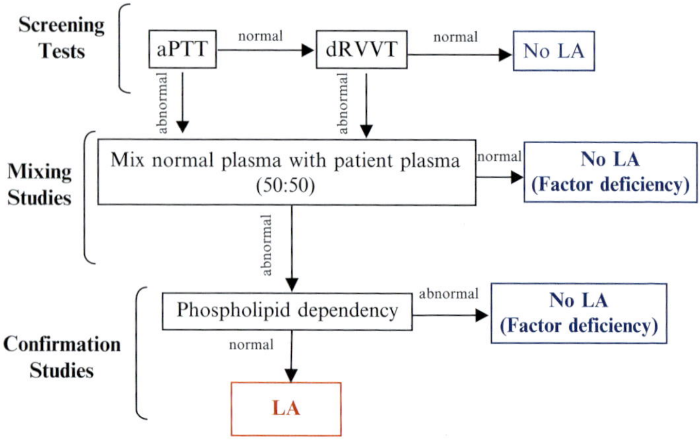

FIG. 3.2. Algorithm for the detection of lupus anticoagulant (LA).

predicting thrombosis, differentiating pathogenic (autoimmune) from nonpathogenic (infection or drug-induced) antibodies, since β2GPI is an absolute requirement for binding of autoimmune aCL to cardiolipin in ELISA. This molecule has five distinct domains. The phospholipid-binding site is present within the fifth domain of β2GPI (Fig. 3.3). Early studies suggested that the epitope for aCL binding was located in the fourth domain. However, current experimental evidence supports the idea that the major epitopes are contained in domain I.

Clinical studies of anti-β2GPI ELISAs suggest that positivity in these assays is more closely associated with clinical manifestations of the antiphospholipid syndrome (APS) than positivity in conventional aCL ELISAs. This is predominantly due to enhanced diagnostic specificity; although anti-β2GPI

→

FIG. 3.3. Structure of human β2-GPI and binding model of β2-GPI and phospholipids. (**a**) Two views, related by 180° rotation of the electrostatic potential surface of β2-GPI. (**b**) Positively charged patch on the aberrant half of domain V. (**c**) Diagram of the proposed model for binding of β2-GPI to anionic phospholipids. From Khamashta 2000, with kind permission from Springer [Reprinted from Bouma et al. 1999].

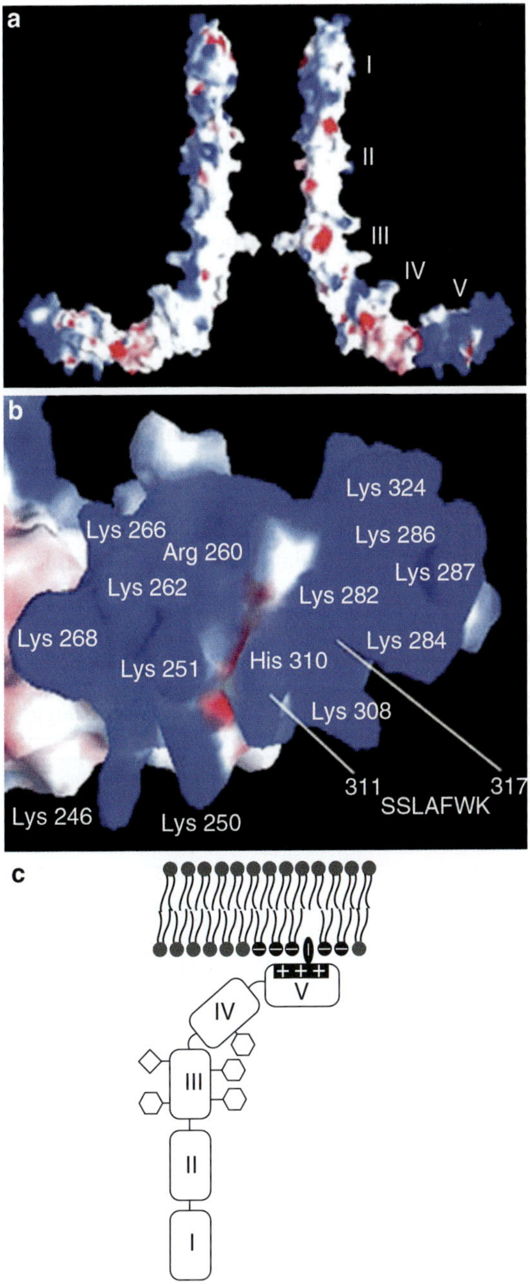
a
I
II
III
IV
V
b
Lys 324
Lys 266
Lys 286
Arg 260
Lys 287
Lys 262
Lys 282
Lys 268
Lys 284
His 310
Lys 251
Lys 308
311
317
SSLAFWK
Lys 246
Lys 250
c
IV
V
III
II
I

assays have also identified a small number of patients who have clinical manifestations of the APS, but are negative in conventional aPL assays.

3.3.2 Antiprothrombin Antibodies

Prothrombin is a 72 kD single-chain glycoprotein with 579 amino acid residues, three carbohydrate chains, and ten γ-carboxyglutamic acid residues (Fig. 3.4). Prothrombin is the prime contributor to the blood coagulation process that becomes activated to thrombin by the tenase complex formed by factor Xa and factor V in the presence of calcium and phospholipids. This activation reaction subsequently triggers fibrinogen polymerization to fibrin.

Prothrombin is a major phospholipid-binding protein, which was first reported to be a cofactor for LA in 1959. Antiprothrombin antibodies are detected by ELISA using PT coated onto irradiated plates (aPT), or in complex with PS

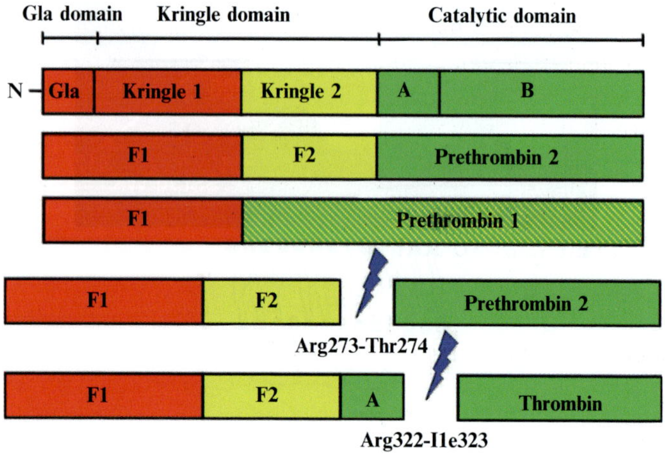

FIG. 3.4. Schematic representation of the prothrombin molecule cleavage at Arg273–Thr274 results in the liberation of prothrombin fragment 1+2 (residues 1–273) and prethrombin 2 (residues 274–581); further cleavage at Arg322–Ile323 results in the formation of α-thrombin.

(aPS-PT). In our experience, antiprothrombin antibodies are frequently found in patients with SLE, and their presence is associated with thrombosis. More significantly, 48% of the patients with aPL-related clinical features who werere negative for standard tests had antiprothrombin antibodies, making these antibodies potential markers for the APS.

Anti-β2GPI and antiprothrombin antibodies both have LA effects. Thus, one might expect that ELISA assays specifically measuring each single antibody should offer an advantage over clotting tests, which give only a qualitative estimate of an in vitro phenomenon, or that at least they are comparable in their correlations with clinical outcomes. Two recent systematic reviews, however, do not provide support for the replacement of coagulation tests with ELISAs and this remains an area of debate.

3.3.3 Other Specificities

A variety of antibodies directed to other plasma proteins such as protein C, protein S, annexin V, and factor XII have been reported in patients with APS. However, the clinical significance of these antibodies is unclear, and they are not being tested routinely.

3.4 Antiphospholipid Antibodies as Diagnostic Markers

Laboratory diagnosis of APS relies on the demonstration of a positive aCL antibody or anti-β2GPI test by an in-house or commercially available enzyme-linked immunosorbent assay (ELISA), or on the presence of LA by a coagulation-based test (Fig. 3.5). It is important that both tests are performed in patients suspected of having APS. Persistence of the positive tests must be demonstrated and other causes and underlying factors considered. The aCL test is positive in about 80% of patients with APS, the LA test is positive in about 20%, and

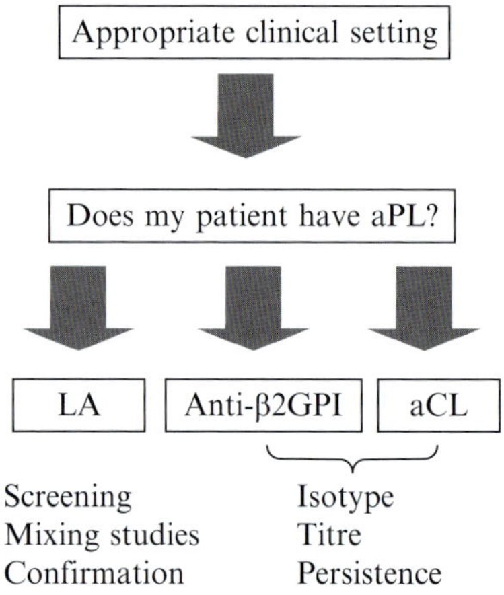

FIG. 3.5. Algorithm for the diagnosis of APS.

both are positive in about 60% of cases. Even though there is a strong correlation between aCL and anti-β2GPI, antibodies to β2GPI have also been described as the sole aPL in some cases.

3.5 Indications for aPL Testing

aPL should be tested routinely in all patients who are newly diagnosed with an autoimmune connective tissue disease especially SLE or Sjögren's syndrome, since the prevalence of aPL in these disorders ranges between 30 and 50%. The finding of aPL at disease onset may have significant consequences later in the disease course in terms of predicting morbidity and mortality. Patients who suffer thrombotic events at relatively young age should also be considered for testing. Patients with stroke, myocardial infarction, and venous thrombosis under the age of 50 may be at risk of further thrombotic events if they are aPL positive. Similarly, women with pregnancy morbidity, including miscarriage, fetal death, intra-uterine growth restriction, intra-uterine death/still-birth, pregnancy-induced hypertension, pre-eclampsia, and eclampsia, should also have aPL measured. There is a wide spectrum of aPL-related pregnancy morbidity.

As some data suggest that aPL may be "consumed" during a thrombotic episode, it should be measured between 6 weeks and 3 months postthrombosis to confirm the results. Steroid therapy and the development of the nephrotic syndrome may also be associated with a false-negative result.

A recent study has suggested that aPL may appear many years prior to the diagnosis of an autoimmune connective tissue disease such as lupus, and aPL-positive patients appeared to be at risk of more severe lupus later in the disease course, suggesting that immune dysregulation leading to autoantibody production may precede the appearance of symptoms by many years.

References

Amengual O, Atsumi T, Khamashta MA, Koike T, Hughes GRV (1996) Specificity of ELISA for antibody to beta 2-glycoprotein I in patients with antiphospholipid syndrome. Br J Rheumatol 35(12):1239–1243

Bertolaccini ML, Hughes GR (2006) Antiphospholipid antibody testing: which are most useful for diagnosis? Rheum Dis Clin North Am 32(3):455–463

Bertolaccini ML, Sanna G, Ralhan S, Gennari LC, Merrill JT, Khamashta MA et al (2003) Antibodies directed to protein S in patients with systemic lupus erythematosus: prevalence and clinical significance. Thromb Haemost 90(4):636–641

Bertolaccini ML, Hughes GR, Khamashta MA (2004) Revisiting antiphospholipid antibodies: from targeting phospholipids to phospholipid binding proteins. Clin Lab. 50(11–12):653–665

Bertolaccini ML, Atsumi T, Koike T, Hughes GR, Khamashta MA (2005) Antiprothrombin antibodies detected in two different assay systems. Prevalence and clinical significance in systemic lupus erythematosus. Thromb Haemost 93(2):289–297

Bertolaccini ML, Mepani K, Sanna G, Hughes GR, Khamashta MA (2007) Factor XII autoantibodies as a novel marker for thrombosis and adverse obstetric history in patients with systemic lupus erythematosus. Ann Rheum Dis 66(4):533–536

Bouma B et al (1999) Adhesion mechanism of human beta(2)-glycoprotein I to phospholipids based on its crystal structure. EMBO J 18:5166–5174

Brandt JT, Triplett DA, Alving B, Scharrer I (1995) Criteria for the diagnosis of lupus anticoagulants: an update. On behalf of the Subcommittee on Lupus anticoagulant/Antiphospholipid Antibody of the Scientific and Standardisation Committee of the ISTH. Thromb Haemost 74:1185–1190

de Laat B, Derksen RH, Urbanus RT, de Groot PG (2005) IgG antibodies that recognize epitope Gly40-Arg43 in domain I of beta 2-glycoprotein I cause LAC, and their presence correlates strongly with thrombosis. Blood 105(4):1540–1545

de Laat B, Derksen RH, van Lummel M, Pennings MT, de Groot PG (2006) Pathogenic anti-beta2-glycoprotein I antibodies recognize domain I of beta2-glycoprotein I only after a conformational change. Blood 107(5):1916–1924

Khamashta MA (2000) Hughes syndrome: antiphospholipid syndrome. Springer, London, p 474

Chapter 4
Classification Criteria for APS

An international consensus statement on classification criteria for definite APS was published in 1999. A patient with APS must meet at least one of the two clinical criteria (vascular thrombosis or pregnancy complications) and at least one of the two laboratory criteria (aCL and/or LA). Although these criteria have been shown to be specific and sensitive for the classification of primary and secondary APS, the absence of "major" or "essential" features in the presence of "minor" features should not discourage the clinician from making the diagnosis when other causes of such features have been ruled out, since other well-recognized features of APS such as thrombocytopenia, hemolytic anemia, transient ischemic attacks, transverse myelitis, livedo reticularis, valvular heart disease, demyelinating syndromes, chorea, and migraine were not thought to have as strong an association as the final criteria and were excluded as classification criteria. These criteria have been revised in 2006 to include anti-β2GPI as a laboratory criterion for APS, and laboratories around the world are being encouraged to standardize their methodology for the detection of these antibodies (Table 4.1).

M.L. Bertolaccini et al., *Antiphospholipid Syndrome Handbook*, DOI 10.1007/978-1-84628-735-0_4,

TABLE 4.1. 2006 preliminary criteria for the classification of definite antiphospholipid syndrome.

Clinical criteria
Vascular thrombosis: ≥ one arterial, venous, or small vessel thrombosis in any tissue or organ, confirmed by imaging or histopathology in the absence of significant evidence of inflammation in the vessel wall
Pregnancy morbidity
≥One unexplained death of a morphologically normal fetus at or beyond the tenth week of gestation
≥One premature births of a morphologically normal neonate at or beyond the 34th week of gestation, due to severe preeclampsia, eclampsia, or placental insufficiency
≥Three unexplained consecutive spontaneous abortions before the tenth week of gestation (maternal anatomic or hormonal abnormalities and chromosomal causes excluded)
Laboratory criteria[b]
Medium or high titers of IgG and/or IgM aCL measured by a standardized ELISA for β2-glycoprotein I-dependent aCL
A positive lupus anticoagulant test, detected according to the guidelines of the ISTH (38)
Anti-β2GPI of IgG and/or IgM isotype in serum or plasma (in titre >99th percentile)

[a]Definite APS is considered to be present if at least one clinical and one laboratory criteria are met

[b]Positivity should be present on two or more occasions at least 12 weeks apart for any of the tests

References

Miyakis S, Lockshin MD, Atsumi T, Branch DW, Brey RL, Cervera R et al (2006) International consensus statement on an update of the classification criteria for definite antiphospholipid syndrome (APS). J Thromb Haemost 4(2):295–306

Wilson WA, Gharavi AE, Koike T, Lockshin MD, Branch DW, Piette JC et al (1999) International consensus statement on preliminary classification criteria for definite antiphospholipid syndrome: report of an international workshop. Arthritis Rheum 42(7):1309–1311

Chapter 5
Mortality, Morbidity, and Damage Associated with aPL

APS has a significant impact on survival. In 10 years, up to 50% of the aPLs positive patients may develop the syndrome, around 59% may experience a recurrent thrombosis with a mortality of around 10%. The most common thrombotic events are cerebrovascular accidents (11.8%), coronary occlusions (7.4%), and pulmonary emboli (5.9%).

There is an increasing evidence that thrombosis contributes to irreversible organ damage as well as mortality in lupus patients with aPL.

References

Ruiz-Irastorza G, Egurbide MV, Ugalde J, Aguirre C (2004) High impact of antiphospholipid syndrome on irreversible organ damage and survival of patients with systemic lupus erythematosus. Arch Intern Med 164(1):77–82

Shah NM, Khamashta MA, Atsumi T, Hughes GRV (1998) Outcome of patients with anticardiolipin antibodies: a 10 year follow-up of 52 patients. Lupus 7(1):3–6

M.L. Bertolaccini et al., *Antiphospholipid Syndrome Handbook*,
DOI 10.1007/978-1-84628-735-0_5,

Chapter 6
Differences Between Primary and Secondary APS

In general, there are no significant differences in the cardinal clinical features of APS such as arterial or venous thrombosis or pregnancy morbidity whether the syndrome is primary or secondary to an underlying connective tissue disorder. IgM aCLs are more commonly seen in SLE than PAPS but there is no difference in thrombotic rates.

The distinction between PAPS and APS due to SLE can sometimes be difficult. In both the conditions, thrombocytopenia, anemia, renal, and central nervous system disease may be seen. Anti-dsDNA or antibodies to extractable nuclear antigens are not found in PAPS, and their presence usually suggests SLE as a secondary cause. The number of cases reported in the literature of patients with PAPS evolving into SLE is small, and some patients have developed the disease after 10 years. The presence of high titre ANA (>1:320), low complement levels, and lymphopenia may be predictive.

References

Gomez-Puerta JA, Martin H, Amigo MC, Aguirre MA, Camps MT, Cuadrado MJ et al (2005) Long-term follow-up in 128 patients with primary antiphospholipid syndrome: do they develop lupus? Medicine (Baltimore) 84(4):225–230

M.L. Bertolaccini et al., *Antiphospholipid Syndrome Handbook*,
DOI 10.1007/978-1-84628-735-0_6,

Vianna JL, Khamashta MA, Ordi-Ros J, Font J, Cervera R, Lopez-Soto A et al (1994) Comparison of the primary and secondary antiphospholipid syndrome: a European Multicenter Study of 114 patients. Am J Med 96(1):3–9

Chapter 7
Clinical Features

7.1 Central Nervous System Involvement

Central nervous system (CNS) involvement is one of the most prominent clinical manifestations of APS (Table 7.1). Neurological manifestations were only second to venous thrombosis in a prospective cohort of 1,000 patients with APS published by the Euro-Phospholipid Project Group.

The mechanism of neurological involvement in patients with APS is thought to be primarily thrombotic in origin. However, there are many neuropsychiatric syndromes, where no structural lesions are evident in imaging studies of brain, suggesting aPL-mediated mechanisms other than thrombosis may be playing a role, such as aPL direct effect on neurons, glia, and myelin.

7.1.1 Cerebral Ischemia

Cerebral ischemic disease associated with aPL is the most common arterial thrombotic manifestation. Stroke and transient ischemic attacks (TIAs) are considered the second most common clinical manifestations of APS after venous trombosis (Fig. 7.1). *Moreover*, in the European Working Party on systemic lupus erythematosus (SLE) (which studied a cohort of 1,000 patients with SLE), thromboses were the most common cause of death during follow up and were always

M.L. Bertolaccini et al., *Antiphospholipid Syndrome Handbook*,
DOI 10.1007/978-1-84628-735-0_7,

TABLE 7.1. Neuropsychiatric manifestations associated with aPL.

Cerebrovascular disease:
Stroke
TIA
Cerebral venous sinus thrombosis
Acute ischemic encephalopathy
Chorea
Atypical migrainous-like events
Seizures
Headache
Multiple sclerosis-like syndrome
Idiopathic intracranial hypertension
Transverse myelopathy
Other neurological syndromes:
Sensorineural hearing loss (sudden or progressive)
Guillain-Barré Syndrome
Transient global amnesia
Ocular syndromes (Amaurosis fugax, ischemic optic neuropathy, vaso-occlusive retinopathy)
Dystonia-Parkinsonism
Progressive supra-nuclear palsy
Diabetic peripheral neuropathy
Orthostatic hypotension
Cognitive dysfunction
Dementia
Psychiatric disorders (depression, psychosis)

associated with APS. The most common thrombotic events in these patients were strokes (11.8%), followed by myocardial infarction (7.4%) and pulmonary embolism (5.9%). The risk of recurrent stroke appears to have increased in APS patients.

The average age of onset of aPL-associated cerebral ischemia is several decades younger than the typical cerebral ischemia in the general population. Thus, aPL should be included in the investigation of all individuals under 50 with stroke.

Cerebral ischemic events can occur in any vascular territory, but in general, the territory of the middle cerebral artery (MCA) is more affected, mainly due to local thrombosis (Fig. 7.2).

Cardiac emboli may be another cause of cerebral ischemia in patients with aPL. In fact, the prevalence of valvular

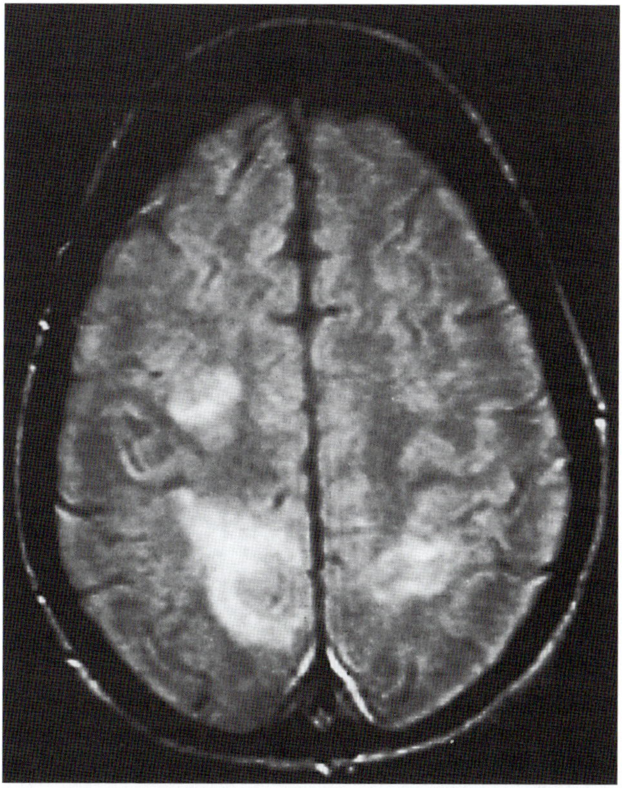

FIG. 7.1. Brain magnetic resonance imaging (MRI) study showing multiple strokes in a young woman with antiphospholipid antibodies, strokes, and seizures, from Khamashta 2000, with kind permission from Springer.

anormalities, particularly left side valve lesions, is higher in SLE and APS *(see cardiac manifestations, valvular disease)*. Another possible emboli source can be the heart chambers themselves or the internal carotid artery.

An ischemic stroke can be isolated or multiple and recurrent. Episodes of cerebral ischemia, mainly focal, can be transient or permanent. Amaurosis fugax, transient paresthesias, motor weakness, vertigo, and transient global ischemia can

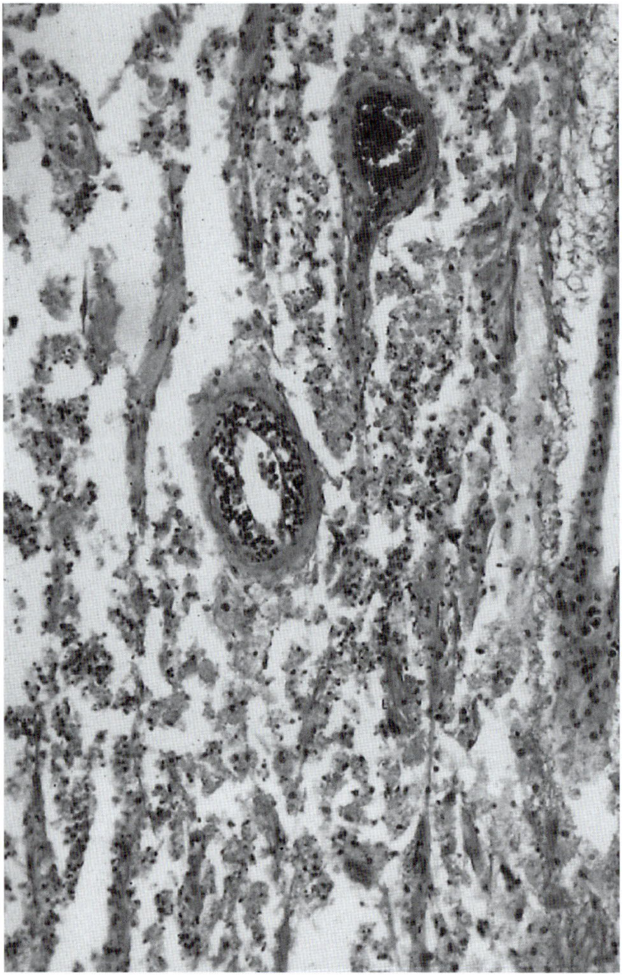

Fig. 7.2. Hematoxalin and esosin-stained section of postmortem brain tissue from a patient with aPL and the catastrophic antiphospholipid antibody syndrome. *Arrow* indicates a small cerebral blood vessel with thrombus, but no inflammation, from Khamashta 2000, with kind permission from Springer.

all be expressions of TIAs. A chronic multifocal disease can produce multi-infarct dementia.

7.1.2 Subcortical High-Intensity Lesions on Brain MRI

Brain MRI in aPL patients with ischemic stroke typically shows cortical abnormalities consistent with large vessel occlusion. However small sub-cortical white matter high-density lesions on brain MRI are frequently found in patients with aPL, and also in SLE patients with or without overt neuropsychiatric manifestations (Fig. 7.3). The finding of these lesions may represent a diagnostic and therapeutic dilemma especially in young patients. The significance of these lesions is not completely understood. They are often defined as consistent with the presence of small vessel disease by the neuroradiologists. It has been suggested that they may be due to multiple small infarcts. There is evidence that the presence of similar lesions is associated with a higher risk for stroke, seizures, psychiatric disturbances, dementia, and cognitive disorders.

In case of a patient with neurologic manifestations with cortical or subcortical high-intensity lesions, long-term oral anticoagulation (INR 3–4) should be considered.

7.1.3 Epilepsy

Several studies have proved the direct association between aPL and seizures in SLE patients, even excluding cerebrovascular accidents (an important cause of epilepsy).

The paper published by the Euro-Phospholipid Project Group (Cervera et al., 2002) reported seizures in 7% of 1,000 patients with APS. Shoenfeld et al. reported epilepsy in 8.6% of 538 patients with APS. Epilepsy was more prevalent among patients with APS secondary to SLE (13.7%) when compared to those with PAPS (6%).

Different forms of seizures are seen in association with aPL and all ages may be affected. Epilepsy should be treated with antiepileptic drugs.

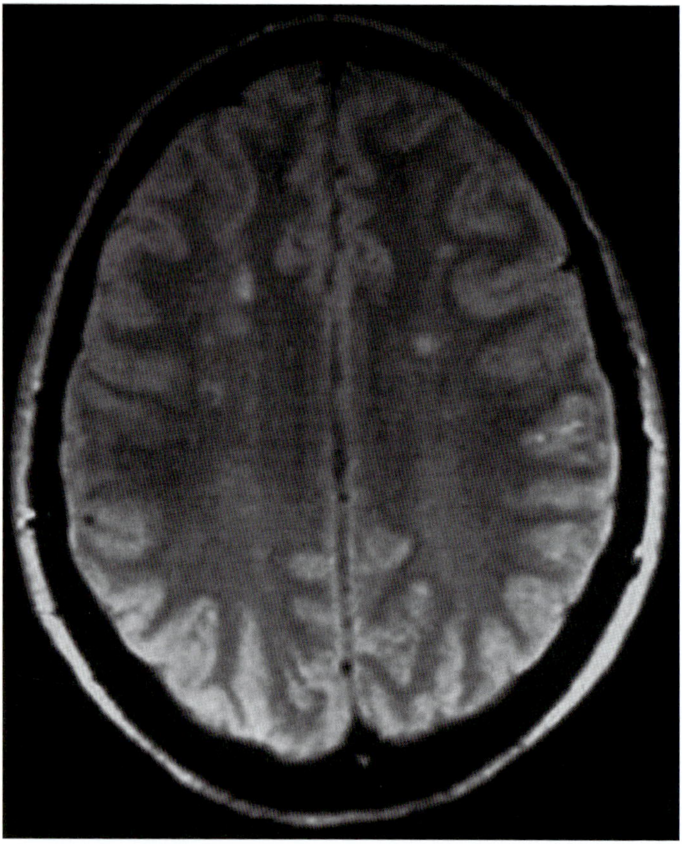

FIG. 7.3. White matter hyperintensity lesions (WMHL) MRI scan.

7.1.4 Multiple Sclerosis-Like Syndrome

Clinical syndromes mimicking multiple sclerosis (MS), mainly in its relapsing-remitting pattern, are reported to occur in association with aPL. Laboratory findings and MRI studies are not often useful tools to distinguish APS from MS. With regard to the MRI, large size lesions and their atypical topographic distribution in aPL patients. Brain MRI may be consistent with demyelination and sometimes difficult to differentiate from MRI pictures in MS. Therefore, differential diagnosis may be difficult, and some APS patients can be misdiagnosed as having MS.

A careful interview of the patient, a past medical history of thrombotic events, and pregnancy morbidity in female patients may be useful in the differential diagnosis, favoring APS. The abruptness of onset and resolution of symptoms, especially in regard to visual symptoms, and atypical neurological features for MS such as headache or epilepsy, strongly suggest APS rather than MS. Evoked potential studies have been proposed as a good tool to differentiate both disorders.

If not all, at least a subgroup of patients with "nonclassic" MS should be tested for aPL. If high suspicion, management should include antiplatelet or even anticoagulant agents.

7.1.5 Headache

One of the most prominent features in patients with APS is headache. This symptom, a common complaint of APS patients in clinical practice, can vary from classic intermittent migraine to almost continuous incapacitating headache. The association of migraine and aPL is controversial with widely varying results from different series.

One of the major problems is that headaches, often nonmigrainous, have been loosely termed "migraine," and these headaches may precede or accompany TIAs or CVAs.

The available data suggest an association between the migraine-like phenomena and aPL, but not between migraine headache and aPL. Thus, aPL should be included in the investigation of all young individuals with migraine irresponsive to conventional treatment.

With regard to the treatment, it usually responds to conventional therapy. In some cases it has been reported to improve remarkably with low-dose aspirin; very resistant cases may require heparin or warfarin as alternative therapy.

7.2 Cardiac Manifestations

Around 40% of patients with APS may develop cardiac manifestations, but significant morbidity appears in less than 10% of these patients (Table 7.2).

7.2.1 Valvular Disease

Heart valve lesions are the most common cardiac manifestations described in patients with aPL. According to a review performed by Nesher et al., 36% of PAPS patients and 35% of SLE patients had valvulopathy. The same review showed that 48% of aPL-positive SLE patients had valvulopathy, compared with only 21% of aPL-negative SLE patients. Although most cases are symptomless, some cases evolve to severe valvular dysfunction resulting in cardiac failure, sometimes requiring valve replacement.

Thickening of the valve leaflets is the most common lesion detected by echocardiography in both SLE and PAPS patients (Fig. 7.4). The mitral valve is involved most commonly, followed by the aortic valve. Most thickened valves develop hemodynamic abnormalities, occurring roughly in 25% of all patients with SLE or PAPS. The pathogenesis of valvular abnormalities in APS is not entirely clear. It has been postulated that

Table 7.2. Cardiac manifestations in APS.

Valves:
Leaflet thickening (the most frequent)
Vegetations (Libman-Sacks endocarditis)
Stenosis
Regurgitation
Coronary arteries:
Ischemic heart disease: Myocardial Infarction, Angina, Cardiac Syndrome X.
Coronary bypass graft and angioplasty occlusions.
Other:
Intracardiac thrombus
Acute/chronic cardiomyopathy (due to microangiopathy)

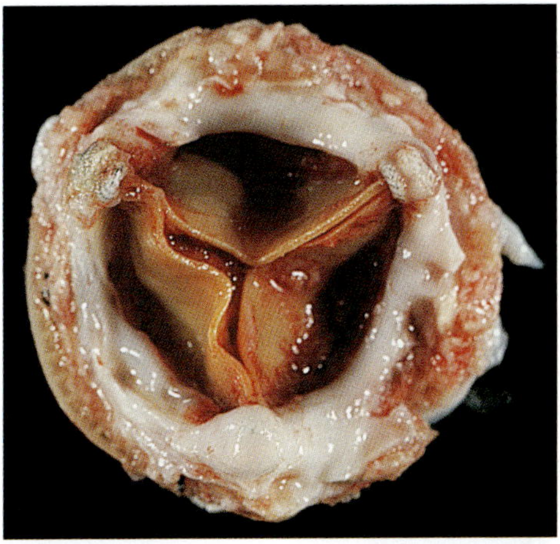

FIG. 7.4. Valvular thickening and thrombosis in a prosthetic mitral valve of a patient. With primary APS, from Khamashta 2000, with kind permission from Springer.

aPL could cause straightforward valvular or endothelial injury unrelated to clinical severity of the disease.

Most cases are clinically silent and detected by either chest auscultation, echocardiography, or at autopsy. Nevertheless, 5% of all SLE and APS patients develop severe mitral or aortic regurgitation (with symptoms such as fatigue, shortness of breath, and orthopnea), and valve replacement surgery is required in half of these patients.

Although infective endocarditis has been described in several patients with SLE, it is a very uncommon complication of this disease. However, several SLE patients have been reported presenting with the following combination of signs and serology: (1) fever, (2) cardiac murmurs with echocardiographic demonstration of valve vegetations, (3) splinter hemorrhages (Fig. 7.5), (4) serological evidence of SLE activity (e.g., high titers of antibodies to dsDNA and low serum complement levels), (5) moderate to high elevations of aPL, and (6) repeatedly culture-negative blood samples. All these manifestations are explicable on the basis of SLE activity and complications associated with the APS.

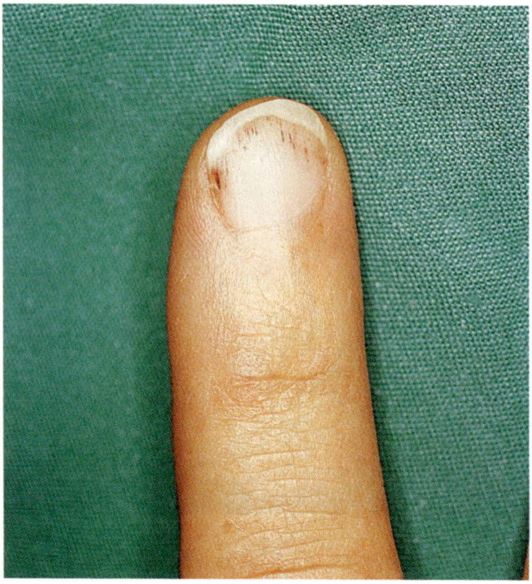

FIG. 7.5. Splinter hemorrhages in a patient with valve vegetations and aPL, from Khamashta 2000, with kind permission from Springer.

A further problem in patients with aPL and valve lesions is the development of embolic cerebrovascular complications. High levels of IgG aCL has been associated with the development of severe valvular regurgitation and with a high incidence of valvular surgery and thromboembolic events.

With regard to long-term treatment, it is of note that anticoagulant or antiaggregant therapy does not contribute to the disappearance of vegetations or other valve lesions, and data about response to corticosteroids are contradictory. Moreover, surgical excision of uninfected valvular vegetations may not prevent recurrence. Nevertheless, prophylactic antiplatelet therapy may be amend to asymptomatic patients, while anticoagulation may be the best choice for patients with valvulopathy who have had any evidence of thromboembolic disease. In some cases, valvular damage may result in significant hemodynamic compromise, requiring surgery and further full anticoagulation.

7.2.2 Coronary Artery Disease

Accelerated atherosclerosis in SLE, besides classical risk factors, such as age, sex, smoking, hyperlipidemia, hypertension, diabetes, hyperhomocysteinemia, cronic renal insufficiency, obesity, is related to a permanent pro-inflammatory state, long-term steroid administration and aPL.

The prevalence of aPL in patients with myocardial infarction seems to be between 5 and 15%. Elevated levels of aCL imply an increased risk for the development of myocardial infarction and recurrent cardiac events. Similar data have been described for angina.

A correlation between the levels of aCL and antibodies to oxidized LDL (anti-oxLDL) , as well as the cumulative effect of both for the risk of myocardial infarction, has been described. Anti-oxLDL antibodies have been considered as markers of atherosclerosis.

In the same way, among patients with significant aCL there is a substantial failure rate following aortocoronary venous bypass grafting, as well as high restenosis rate after percutaneous transluminal coronary angioplasty (PTCA).

Therefore, aPL general screening of ischemic cardiac disease patients is not indicated, but should be requested in case of:

- Younger patients (age <50)
- Those with a previous history of venous or arterial thrombosis or recurrent fetal losses
- Those with a family history of an autoimmune disease (especially lupus)

Long-term anticoagulation is indicated in cases of aPL-related coronary artery disease.

7.3 Skin Manifestations

Several skin manifestations have been described in patients with APS (Table 7.3). The most frequent skin lesions are livedo reticularis and skin ulcers.

TABLE 7.3. Skin manifestations in APS.

Livedo reticularis
Ulcers
Necrotizing vasculitis
Livedoid vasculitis
Cutaneous gangrene
Superficial thromphlebitis
Pseudovasculitis lesions: nodules, papules, pustules, palmar-plantar erythema
Splinter hemorrhage
Anetoderma

Around 40% of patients with APS begin their disease with skin manifestations, and 40% of them will develop multisystem thrombotic phenomena during the course of the disease. However, it is hard to predict if the patient who only has a skin lesion will later develop an extra cutaneous thrombotic event. Thus, the presence of multiple subungual hemorrhages might coincide with thrombotic events of other organs such as the brain, skin, adrenal glands, kidney, etc.

Skin necrosis and digital ischemia should be considered as major thrombotic events (Fig. 7.6); in these cases, patients should receive long-term anticoagulant treatment. The approach to minor skin manifestations is less clear. It is yet to be defined whether platelet antiaggregation is enough or whether it will be necessary to use more aggressive treatments, such as anticoagulation.

Although anecdotal, alternative successful treatments have been proposed for patients resistant to standard approaches, such as sildenafil or intravenous infusion of recombinant tissue plasminogen activator in the treatment of nonhealing ulcers.

7.3.1 Livedo Reticularis

Livedor reticularis is the most common skin manifestation in patients with APS (Fig. 7.7). It may be the presenting sign of APS in 15–40%, and may be seen in up to 70% of patients with SLE and APS. It is characterized by a dark purple reticular pattern usually involving the upper and lower limbs.

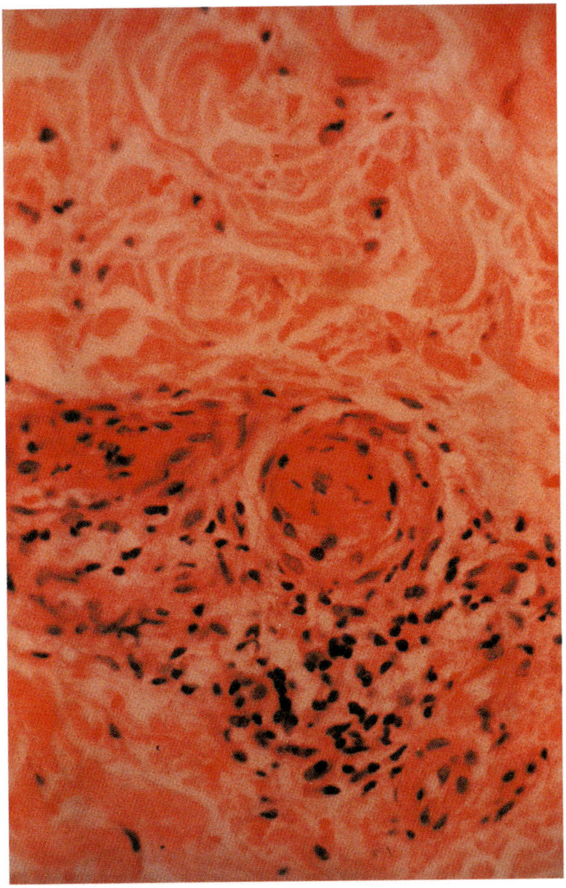

FIG. 7.6. Biopsy of skin with noninflammatory vascular thrombosis (venular) of a patient with SLE and APS, from Khamashta 2000, with kind permission from Springer.

The livid rings are caused by reduced blood flow, and lowered oxygen tension at the peripheries of the skin segments.

Livedo may be observed in normal subjects, especially women, after exposure to cold, displaying a symmetrical and regular mottled pattern. However, the relationship with a large number of pathological conditions is very important

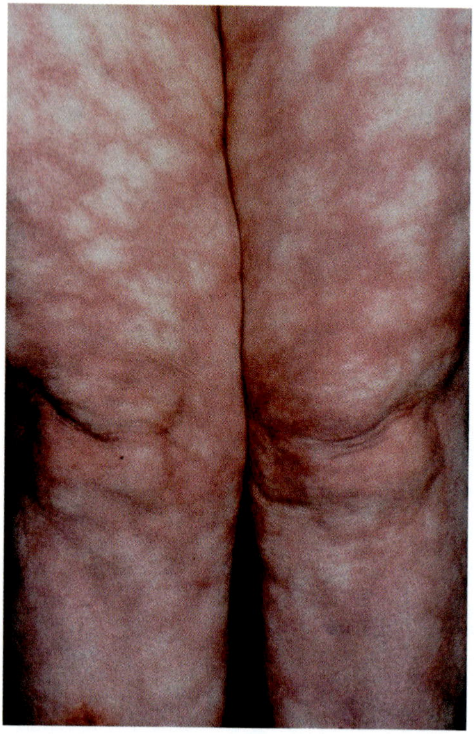

Fig. 7.7. Livedo reticularis.

Table 7.4. Livedo reticularis and associated diseases.

APS
SLE
PAN, cryglobulinemia
Cholesterol embolization
Overlapping syndromes
Sneddon's syndrome
Scleroderma
Drugs: Amantadine
Infectious diseases: Tuberculosis, Syphilis.

(Table 7.4), and it is strongly associated with arterial subset of APS. Pregnancy morbidity has also been frequently observed in patients with livedo.

The association of livedo reticularis with cerebrovascular involvement (known as Sneddon's syndrome) have been accepted as an independent disorder, not clearly associated with aPL.

A detailed examination of the features of the reticular pattern, including location, extension, symmetry, and regularity, and the presence of associated skin lesions will contribute to the differential diagnosis. The pattern of involvement associated with APS is generally disseminated with incomplete circular segments, noninfiltrated, persistent, or irregular with wide ramifications (livedo racemosa). Some patients present a fine, regular, and complete network.

No treatment has proven to be effective for livedo racemosa, which may extend or appear despite anticoagulant or antiplatelet therapy. It is important to reduce or remove other risk factors for thrombosis or arterial wall lesions in view of the higher tendency for stroke and arterial thrombosis in these patients.

7.3.2 Skin Ulcers

Lower limb ulcers are one of the most frequent skin manifestations in patients with APS. They have been observed in 20–30% of these patients (Fig. 7.8).

Although characteristics are variable, ulcers are painful, small (0.5–3.0 cm in diameter), with stellate, oval, or irregular borders surrounded by a purple-brownish, and recurrent purple halo. They are generally located in the ankles, legs, and feet (Fig. 7.9) Healing is usually difficult; when accomplished it results in a white scar with a pigmented halo.

Giant ulcers and cases resembling gangrenous pyoderma have been reported. Postphlebitic ulcers are seldom seen, though an increased prevalence of aPL has been described in elderly patients with venous ulcers.

7.4 Renal Disease

The kidney is a major target organ in APS. Large vessels, both arterial and venous, as well as the intraparenchymatous arteries and microvasculature may all be affected, with different clinical consequences (Table 7.5).

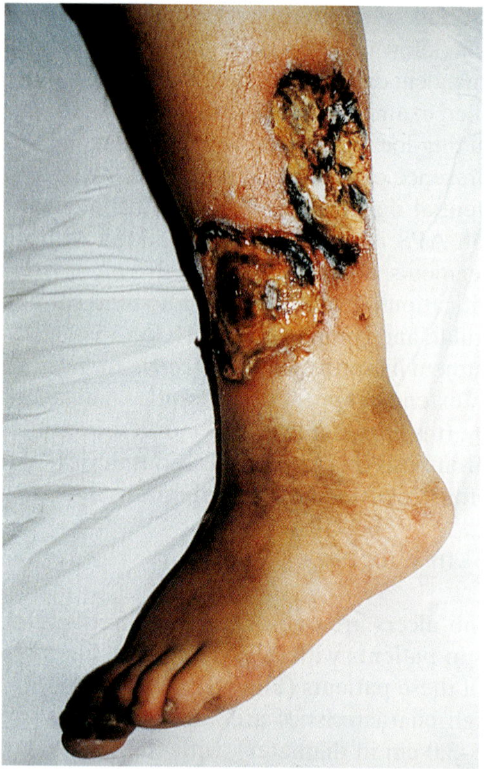

FIG. 7.8. Patient with primary APS that presents necrotic ulcers on the leg and necrosis of the toes, from Khamashta 2000, with kind permission from Springer.

7.4.1 Thrombotic Microangiopathy (TMA)

TMA is the characteristic histologic lesion of the microvasculature in APS-related nephropathy, affecting glomerular capillaries, afferent arterioles, and interlobular arteries (Fig. 7.10). Of course, it is not pathognomonic of APS, as there is a wide range of conditions that present the same histological appearance (Table 7.6).

Depending on the degree and extension of damage, patients could have isolated hypertension (mild to severe), proteinuria

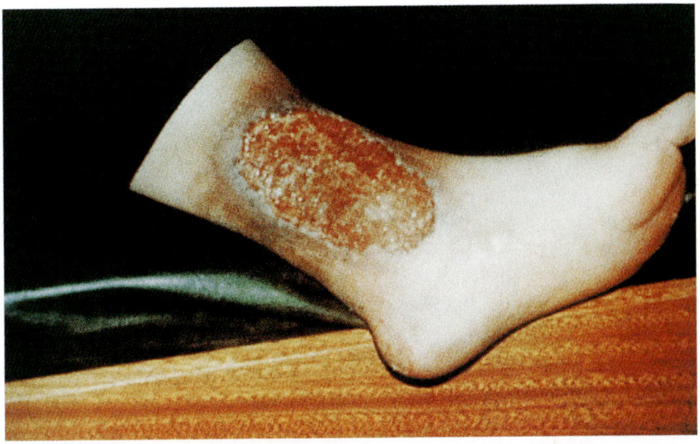

FIG. 7.9. Primary APS with giant skin ulcer on the left leg refractory to anticoagulant and fibrinolytic treatment, from Khamashta 2000, with kind permission from Springer.

TABLE 7.5. Renal vascular involvement in APS.

Vascular lesion	Clinical consequences
Renal artery lesions (thrombosis/occlusion/ stenosis?)	Renovascular hypertension (severe) Renal infarcts (silent, painful, hematuria) Increased likelihood of renal insufficiency
Glomerular capillary thrombosis leading to *glomerular sclerosis* (studied mainly in SLE patients)	Can be observed in up to 40% of aPL negative patients
Renal Thrombotic microangiopathy with/ without cortical necrosis	Systemic hypertension (usually severe) Renal failure (mild to end stage) Proteinuria (mild to nephrotic range) Cortical atrophy
Renal vein thrombosis (uni or bilateral)	Renal failure (if bilateral compromise)

(mild to nephrotic range), and renal failure including cortical necrosis (Fig. 7.11). In fact, APS should be considered in the differential diagnosis of systemic hypertension as APS-related TMA may cause isolated hypertension without significant

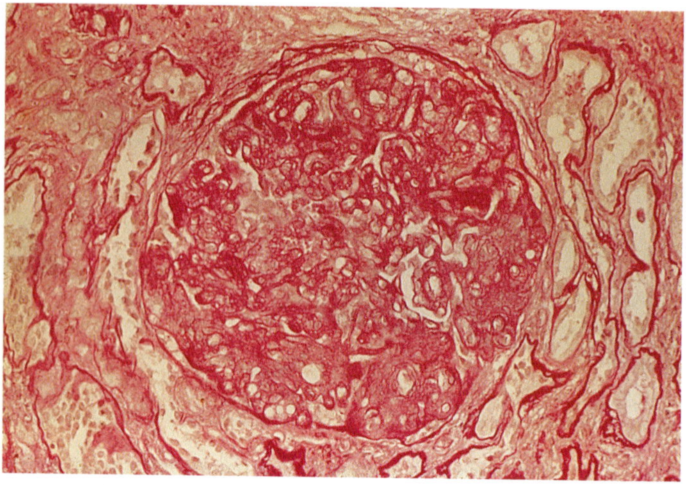

FIG. 7.10. Severe and advanced glomerular thrombotic microangiopathy. Capillary lumina are occluded by severe mesangiolysis and deposition of heterogeneous subendothelial material, leading to a segmental "double contour" aspect (PAS), from Khamashta 2000, with kind permission from Springer.

TABLE 7.6. Other conditions associated with TMA.

Thrombotic thrombocytopenic purpura (TTP)
Hemolytic uremic syndrome (HUS)
Postpartum renal failure
Pre-eclampsia/eclampsia
Scleroderma
Malignant arterial hypertension
Oral contraceptives
Renal transplantation / allograft rejection
Cyclosporine A toxicity
Chemotherapy

renal impartment, as well as in the differential diagnosis of renal damage in patients with SLE and positive aPL.

In chronic cases, fibrosis and focal atrophy, as well as arterial and arteriolar fibromuscular hyperplasia, could be found (Fig. 7.12).

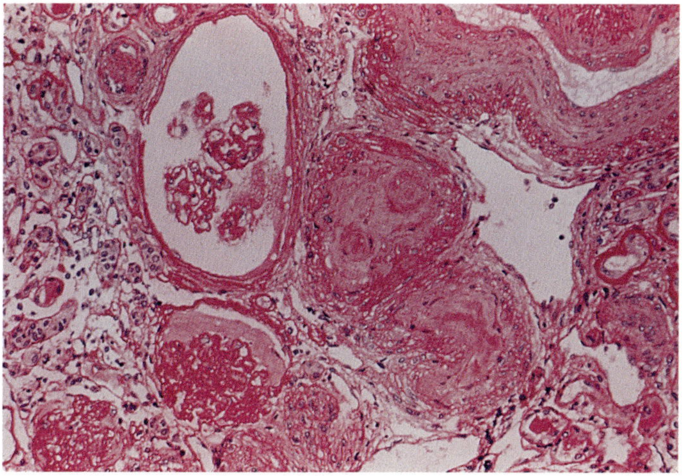

Fig. 7.11. Chronic cortical lesions. There are obsolescent sclerotic glomeruli and a hypoperfused glomerulus with a wide Bowman's space and retracted capillaries. On one of its sides there is a small arteriole with a recanalized thrombus and two lumina. On the other side there are two completely occluded arterioles showing thrombosis, recanalization, and refibrosis. A tortuous arteriole with slightly cellular subendothelial fibrosis is also seen (PAS), from Khamashta 2000, with kind permission from Springer.

7.4.2 Renal Artery Lesions

Large- and medium-size vessel occlusion has been associated with APS. In the presence of aPL, renal infarctions result from partial or total, transient or permanent occlusion of renal arteries (Fig. 7.13). Such occlusions may be caused by diverse mechanisms such as in situ thrombosis/stenosis of a renal artery or an embolic event.

Clinically, severe systemic hypertension, pain in the renal area, hematuria, and renal failure are common forms of presentation of major vessel involvement. On the other hand, arterial hypertension may be labile in early disease, and occasionally, a silent infarct is fortuitously discovered on CT.

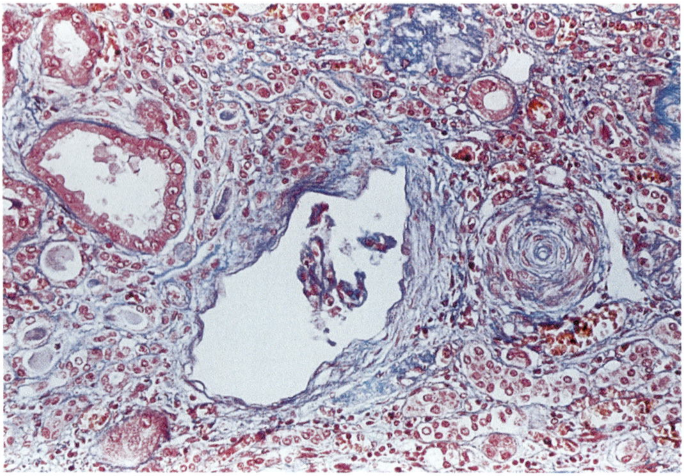

FIG. 7.12. Focal cortical atrophy. There are ischemic glomeruli, an arteriole with "onion skin" hyperplasia of the media, and a "pin point" lumen, generalized tubular atrophy with early dilation in one, and interstitial fibrosis (Masson), from Khamashta 2000, with kind permission from Springer.

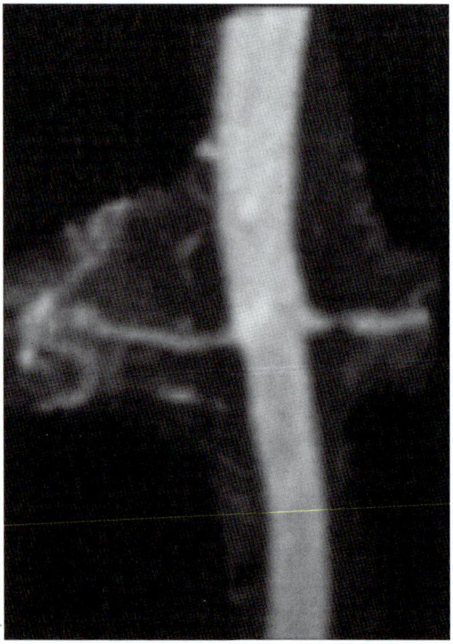

FIG. 7.13. Renal artery stenosis.

Successful treatment with antihypertensive drugs, aspirin, anticoagulant therapy as well as transluminal angioplasty has been reported.

7.4.3 Kidney Transplant

The outcome of kidney transplantation in patients with SLE and end-stage renal failure appears to be similar to that of patients with renal failure from other causes. However, the presence of aPL seems to be associated with a poorer prognosis. Posttransplant thromboembolic phenomena, the recurrence of TMA in the graft despite anticoagulation, and thrombosis of the graft's renal vein have all been reported.

7.5 Hemocytopenia

Thrombocytopenia is one of the most common laboratory abnormalities found in patients with APS. Although less frequently, hemolytic anemia can also be found in APS (Table 7.7). These hemocytopenias are mainly due to autoimmune mechanisms.

7.5.1 Autoimmune Thrombocytopenia

Thrombocytopenia is found in 25–40% of patients with APS, and is one of the most common presenting manifestations. Among these patients, thrombocytopenia is more frequently observed in patients with SLE than in patients with PAPS.

aPL-related thrombocytopenia is a chronic, usually mild and is seldom associated with hemorrhagic complications. Bleeding may be related to several causes other than thrombocytopenia:

Table 7.7. Hematologic disorders in APS.

Autoimmune thrombocytopenia
Autoimmune hemolytic anemia
Microangiopathic hemolytic anemia
Thrombotic thrombocytopenic purpura (TTP)

high-intensity anticoagulation, hypoprothrombinemia (associated with LA), and acquired defects of platelet function often associated with aPL. Values lower than 50×10^9 platelets/L are uncommon, although platelet count can fluctuate with time. Severe thrombocytopenia is an additional risk factor for bleeding complications in these patients. Arterial and/or venous thrombosis in APS may occur despite very low platelet count; however, the frequency of aPL-associated thrombotic events may be lower when platelet count is less than 50×10^9 L.

The pathogenic role for aPL in thrombocytopenia is still controversial. aPL may have a role in thrombocytopenia, but there may be other factors, such as antibodies to platelet membrane glycoproteins, found in 60% of these patients.

7.5.2 Autoimmune Hemolytic Anemia (AIHA)

Hemolytic anemia has been reported in 10% of APS patients; no differences have been found between patients with primary or secondary APS: positive direct Coombs' test has been described in 30–50% of aCL-positive SLE patients, as compared with 2–13% of aCL-negative SLE. However, the association with AIHA is less evident probably due to its relative rareness and the multifactorial origin of anemia in SLE.

Standard treatment of AIHA includes combinations of glucocorticoids, immunosuppressive drugs (such as azathioprine), and splenectomy. Rituximab may be considered prior to splenectomy in some patients.

Evans' syndrome (the clinical association of autoimmune thrombocytopenic purpura with autoimmune hemolytic anemia) has been found in 5% of patients with SLE, mainly in association with high aCL levels, and in 10% of patients with PAPS.

7.6 Obstetric Manifestations

Obstetric complications, together with thrombosis, are the most frequent clinical features of APS (Table 7.8).

Human reproduction is inefficient, with an estimated 50% of conception failing; the majority of these go unrecognized. Approximately 10–15% of pregnancies end in spontaneous abortions prior to 12–14 weeks' gestations (from last menses), most of which are pre-embryonic or embryonic in nature, and 5% of all pregnancies end in pregnancy loss from 14 weeks' gestation through term. Several mechanisms have been proposed in APS (Table 7.9 and 7.10).

There are substantial differences between pregnancy stages (Table 7.11)(Fig. 7.14), and in each stage, pregnancy loss will be determined by different causes (Table 7.12). History taking and obtaining the postmortem findings in previous pregnancy losses are very important (Fig. 7.15). In considering the etiology of first trimester losses, it is also important that obstetricians exclude other relevant causes. It thus seems imperative

TABLE 7.8. Obstetric manifestations associated with APS.

Miscarriages (before 10 weeks)
Fetal death (after 10 weeks)
Pre-eclampsia, eclampsia, and HELLP syndrome
Placental insufficiency (prematurity, fetal growth restriction)
Abruption

TABLE 7.9. Pathogenic mechanisms for pregnancy morbidity in APS.

Placental thrombosis, necrosis and/or infarction
Spiral arterial vasculopathy of decidual vessels
Complement activation
Decreased Annexin V
Acquired protein C resistance

TABLE 7.10. aPL and pregnancy morbidity: proposed mechanisms.

Block placental prostaglandin & thromboxane
Compete with annexin V
Displace annexin V
Inhibit throphoblast proliferation
Block placental gonadotropin

TABLE 7.11. Pregnancy stages.

Pre-embryonic (<4 week after fertilization): implantation and trilaminar pre-embryo with neural axis development.
Embryonic (5–9th weeks of gestation): main organogenesis.
Fetal (from the 10th week until delivery): growth, little organogenesis, and differentiation of formed structures.

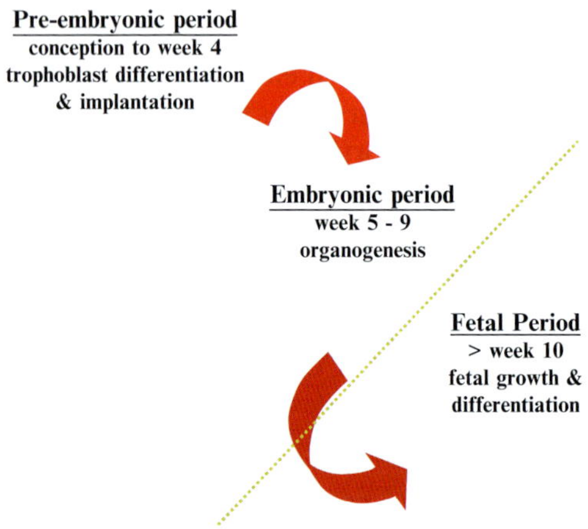

FIG. 7.14. Pregnancy stages.

to assess carefully all cases before aPL can be attributed to be the cause of the pregnancy loss.

Recurrent pregnancy loss (loss of >2 consecutive pregnancies) occurs in an estimated 0.5–1% of women. One previous fetal death increases 5–20 fold the risk to suffer another one. Thorough evaluation of each case is therefore mandatory (Table 7.13).

The pathogenesis of the adverse pregnancy outcome in APS has not yet been fully elucidated although there is active research in this field.

Several studies have proved the strong association between aPL and pregnancy loss. Although in general population early miscarriages (<10 weeks) are the most frequent pregnancy losses, second and third trimester fetal losses are the

TABLE 7.12. Causes of pregnancy loss.

Sporadic miscarriage <10 weeks' gestation
Chromosomal abnormalities of the conceptus/placenta
Fetal loss
Parental structural chromosome abnormalities
Uterine anatomic abnormalities
APS
Thrombophilia, especially factor V Leiden, resistance to activated prot-C, prothrombin 20210 mutation, prot-S deficiency
Intrauterine infection (especially viral)
Alloimmunization to Rh D antigen and other blood group ag
Feto-maternal hemorrhage
Poorly controlled DM
Maternal HTA
Cervical incompetence
Recurrent pre-embryonic or embryonic pregnancy loss
Prenteral structural chromosome abnormalities
Uterine anatomic abnormalities, including congenital malformations
APS
Numeric chromosome abnormalities of the conceptus
Molecular genetic abnormalities of the conceptus or placenta
Hormonal and metabolic disorders
Luteal phase defects
Hypersecretion of luteinizing hormone
Thrombophilia

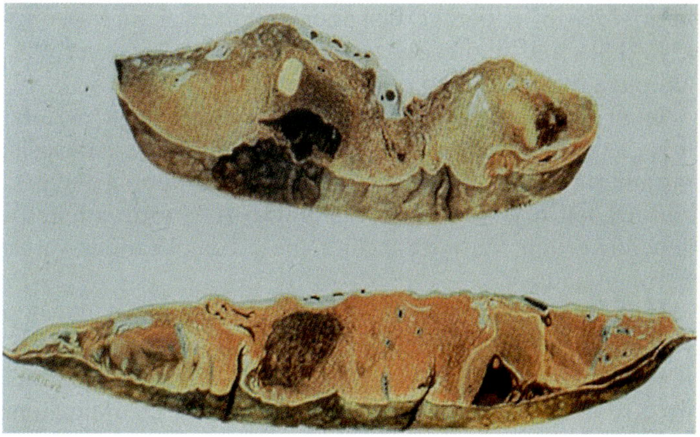

FIG. 7.15. Placental infarction.

TABLE 7.13. Suggested routine evaluation for recurrent pregnancy loss.

History
Pattern and trimester of pregnancy losses and whether a live embryo or fetus was present
Exposure to environmental toxins or drugs
Known gynecologic or obstetric infections
Features associated with APS
Genetic relationship between reproductive partners (consanguinity)
Family history of recurrent miscarriage or syndrome associated with embryonic or fetal loss
Previous diagnostic tests and treatments
Physical
General physical examination
Examination of vagina, cervix and uterus
Tests
Hysterosalpingogram or hysteroscopy
Parental karyotypes
aPL (LA, aCL, anti-β2-glycoprotein1)
Thrombophilia evaluation (factor V Leiden, Prothrombin 20210 mutation)
Luteal phase endometrial biopsy; repeat in next cycle if abnormal
Other lab tests suggested by history and physical examination

most characteristic obstetric complication in APS (present in 50–75% of patients). In patients with SLE and secondary APS, some studies suggest this may be as high as 90%, although this is likely to be an overestimate.

In pregnancies that do not end in miscarriage or fetal loss, there is a high incidence of early onset pre-eclampsia, intrauterine growth restriction, placental abruption, and premature delivery. Because patients with APS form a heterogeneous group, the incidence of these complications varies between units.

It is impossible to predict which women will develop complications in pregnancy, and some women with persistently elevated aPL titers and a history of thromboses and/or thrombocytopenia will have no obstetric complications at all. Previous poor pregnancy outcome remains the most important predictor of future risk.

The strongest relationship between aPL and fetal losses has been found after 14 weeks. Lupus anticoagulant (LA) has shown the strongest association with recurrent fetal losses before 24 weeks' gestation, although it has not been possible to analyze the association of LA with early miscarriages (<13weeks). aCLs are also related with recurrent losses before 24 weeks. IgG aCL is the only one that has been associated with early miscarriages.

Factor V Leiden, the Prothrombin 20210 mutation, and homozygous state for the Homocysteine MTHFR mutation C677T have also been strongly associated with late pregnancy complications and second/third trimester losses.

The physiological changes in the hemostatic system in pregnancy result in an acquired thrombophilic state. In fact, Virchow's triad (venous stasis, hypercoagulability, and vascular damage) occur in the course of uncomplicated pregnancy and delivery.

Pulmonary thromboembolism (PE) remains a major cause of direct maternal mortality, which normally arises from deep venous thrombosis (DVT). PE is more likely to occur postpartum than antepartum, and is strongly associated with cesarean section in epidemiological studies. On the other hand, heritable thrombophilic conditions are found in over 50% of gestational venous thromboembolism.

Women with aPL or obstetric-APS without a history of thrombosis appear to have a substantial high(er) risk of thrombosis during pregnancy and in the postpartum.

7.7 Catastrophic Antiphospholipid Syndrome

Catastrophic APS develops in a minority (<1%) of patients with aPL.It is characterized by acute, life-threatening, diffuse thrombotic microvasculopathy, multiple vascular occlusion, and high titer aPL, with a predilection for kidney, lung, brain, heart, skin, and gastrointestinal tract (Fig. 7.16). Classification criteria for CAPS are shown in Table 7.14.

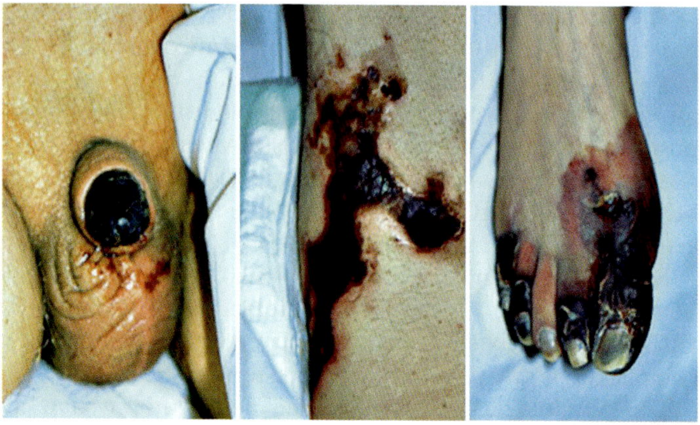

FIG. 7.16. Catastrophic antiphospholipid syndrome.

TABLE 7.14. Preliminary criteria for the classification of catastrophic antiphospholipid antibody syndrome.

Evidence of involvement of three of more organs, systems, or tissues
Development of manifestations simultaneously or in less than a week
Confirmation by histopathology of small-vessel occlusion in at least one organ or tissue[a]
Laboratory confirmation of the presence of antiphospholipid antibodies (lupus anticoagulant or anticardiolipin antibodies)
Definite catastrophic antiphospholipid antibody syndrome
All four criteria
Probable catastrophic antiphospholipid antibody syndrome
All four criteria, except only two organs, systems, or tissues are involved
All four criteria, except for the absence of laboratory confirmation at least 6 weeks apart because of the early death of a patient never previously tested for aPL before the catastrophic event
Criteria 1, 2, and 4
Criteria 1, 3, and 4, and the development of a third event in more than a week, but less than a month, despite anticoagulation

Usually, clinical evidence of vessel occlusions, confirmed by imaging techniques when appropriate. Renal involvement is defined by a 50% rise in serum creatinine, severe systemic hypertension (greater than 190/110 mmHg), or proteinuria (greater than 500 mg per 24 h)

[a]For histopathologic confirmation, significant evidence of thrombosis must be present, although vasculitis may coexist occasionally. If the patient has not been previously diagnosed as having an antiphospholipid antibody syndrome, the laboratory confirmation requires that the presence of antiphospholipid antibodies must be detected on two or more occasions at least 6 weeks apart (not necessarily at the time of the event) according to the proposed clinical criteria for the classification of definite antiphospholipid antibody syndrome

In contrast to the noncatastrophic APS, DVT is uncommon. Roughly, one half of the patients have a prior history of thrombophilia and thrombotic events.

Presentation of the catastrophic APS is often complex as it involves multiple organs concurrently over a short period of time, typically days to weeks (Table 7.15 and 7.16). Fig. 7.17 shows the clinical manifestations attributed to thrombotic events at the time of catastrophic APS.

In two-third of the patients, precipitating factors may have contributed to the development of catastrophic APS. These are included in Table 7.17.

Death occurs in near 50% of patients, and most commonly from cardiac and pulmonary events, predominately from myocardial microthrombi producing cardiac failure, or less often acute myocardial infarction. Respiratory failure especially with ARDS or diffuse alveolar hemorrhage is often a complicating feature in fatal cases.

TABLE 7.15. System involvement in CAPS.

Clinical Manifestations of CAPS
Renal (70%): usually accompanied by hypertension and acute renal failure.
Pulmonary (65%): severe dyspnea, frank adult respiratory distress syndrome (ARDS), pulmonary emboli, sometimes multiple pulmonary infarction, interstitial infiltrates, and intraalveolar hemorrhage.
Central nervous system (55%): major cerebral infarctions, cerebral sinus thrombosis, encephalopathy and seizures.
Cardiac (50%): typical myocardial infarction, diffuse myocardial involvement with congestive heart failure or vale lesions.
Gastrointestinal (45%): vascular occlusions of mesenteric, portal and inferior vena cava, arterial occlusions accompanied by gangrene of the bowels and splenic infarctions, hepatic involvement and pancreatitis.
Skin (40–45%): livedo reticularis, ulcerations, gangrene, purpura, acrocyanosis or digital ischemia.
Other manifestations: adrenal thrombosis, testicular infarction, necrosis of the prostate gland, etc.

TABLE 7.16. Laboratory findings in CAPS.

Laboratory findings
Lupus anticoagulant (80%) or/and *Anticardiolipin antibodies* (85%)
Thrombocytopenia (60%): <100,000/mm
ANA positive (50%)
Hemolytic anemia (25–30%)
Findings consistent with DIC (15–20%): prolonged coagulation tests with increased fibrinogen degradation factors and hypofibrinogenemia.
Schistocytes (15%)

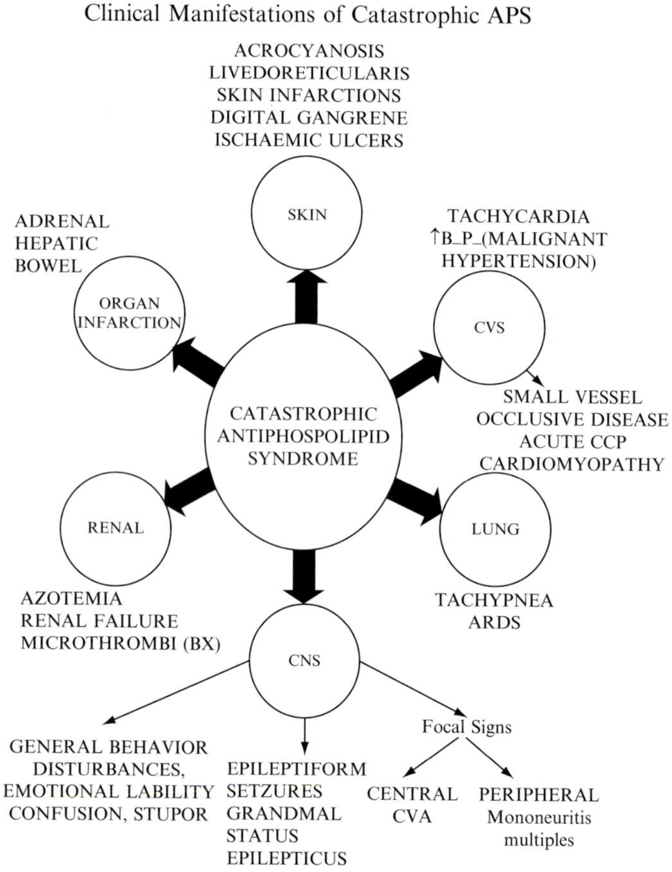

FIG. 7.17. Spectrum of clinical manifestations attributed to thrombotic events at the time of CAPS.

TABLE 7.17. Possible precipitating factors in CAPS.

Infections
Postpartum or recent fetal loss
Minor surgical procedures or surgery
Other: malignancy, medication, anticoagulation withdrawal, and SLE exacerbation.

Surviving an episode of CAPS is typically associated with a good prognosis as only 26% develop further APS-related episodes, but without features of the catastrophic syndrome.

Treatment is empiric and outcomes appear best for patients that received combinations of anticoagulation, steroids, plasmapheresis, intravenous gammaglobulin, and in setting of SLE disease exacerbation, cyclophosphamide.

Treating any precipitating factors, such as prompt use of antibiotics for infection if suspected, and amputation for any necrotic organ are also mandatory.

In 2000, an international registry of patients with CAPS was created by the European Forum on Antiphospholipid Antibodies and can be referenced via the internet at http://www.med.ub.es/MIMMUN/FORUM/CAPS.HTM consisting of nearly 300 patients as of 2008.

7.8 Pulmonary Hypertension

Pulmonary hypertension (PH) is defined as a mean pulmonary artery pressure greater than 25 mmHg, and can be caused by several disorders (Table 7.18). The prevalence of PH has been estimated in 1.8–2% SLE-related APS and in 3.5–5% PAPS. Within APS, PH may result from various causes listed in Table 7.19.

PE is assumed to be the leading cause of PH in APS and its frequency has been ranged in 17–33% of APS patients. The prevalence of aPL in patients with chronic thromboembolic PH has varied between 10 and 20%. The possible role of aPL in the pathophysiology of "unexplained" PH has been proposed, but remains unclear to date.

TABLE 7.18. Conditions associated with pulmonary hypertension.

Arterial pulmonary hypertension (changes in precapillary arteries)
"Primary" arterial PH
Secondary arterial PH (scleroderma, MCTD and other CTD, congenital heart disease, portal hypertension, HIV, anorectic agents, cocaine, etc.)
Postcapillary pulmonary hypertension (changes in pulmonary veins)
Left-sided heart failure
Rarely: pulmonary veno-occlusive disease, pulmonary hemangiomatosis, chronic sclerosing mediastinitis, congenital pulmonary vein anomaly
Proximal pulmonary artery involvement
Mainly: chronic thromboembolic PH
Rarely: metastatic neoplasm, parasites, miscellaneous emboli
Extrinsic vascular compression
Secondary to all chronic causes of hypoxia

TABLE 7.19. Pulmonary hypertension in APS.

APS-related
Pulmonary embolism (acute/chronic)
Left-sided heart failure
Heart valve dysfunction
Myocardial infarction
Myocardiopathy
Portal hypertension
Pulmonary veno-occlusive disease
Not directly APS-related
Chest disorder leading to chronic hypoxia
Fibrosing alveolitis
Coincidental

Evaluation includes careful personal and familial history, complete physical examination, ECG, chest Rx, transesophageal echocardiogram, pulmonary function test with arterial blood gas tension, and additional sleep studies when sleep apnea may be suspected, routine blood tests, liver function tests, complete autoantibody screening including aPL, HIV serology, and either pulmonary angiogram or helicoidal chest CT scan that should be preferred to ventilation-perfusion isotopic scan.

Treatment options are conditioned by the mechanism and cause of PH. However, chronic anticoagulation is needed in all cases, at least to prevent the development of superimposed thrombosis.

When PH results from chronic thromboembolism, inferior vena cava filter may be recommended, and successful thromboendarterectomy has been performed in some patients with very severe disease.

Transplantation, either double-lung, single lung, or heart-lung, may cure the disease, but mortality remains high and donors scarce.

7.9 Systemic Hypertension

The prevalence of hypertension in APS has been described in 30–50% of the patients, depending on the cohort, and seems to be more prevalent in PAPS than in secondary APS. Etipathogenesis is summarized in Table 7.20. Livedo reticularis is a frequent accompanying sign, and has been found in up to 80% of the hypertensive APS patients.

The severity of hypertension varies from mild labile to severe accelerated hypertension.

In case of APS patients with poorly controlled hypertension with antihypertensive drugs, renal artery MRI should be considered to rule out renal artery stenosis.

7.10 Osteoarticular Manifestations

Osteonecrosis and arthralgias are the most frequent manifestations associated with APS (Fig. 7.18). Nontraumatic metatarsal stress fractures have been also described (Fig. 7.19).

TABLE 7.20. Etiopathogenesis of systemic hypertension.

Renal (due to SLE or other associated disease)
Reno-vascular: renal artery stenosis is different from that seen in atherosclerotic disease and fibro-muscular dysplasia.
Thrombotic microangiopathy
Other: obesity, corticosteroids, diabetes mellitus.

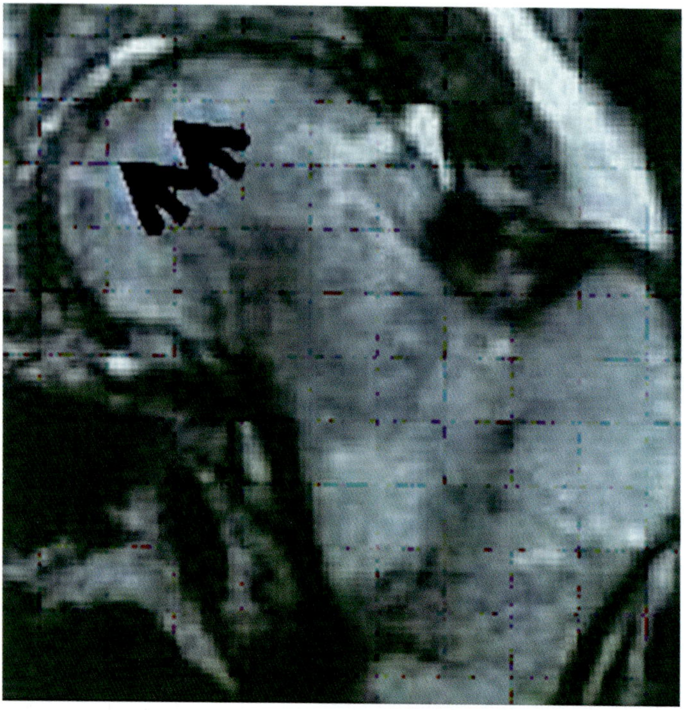

Fig. 7.18. Early osteonecrosis on this T2-weighted spin echo magnetic resonance is indicated by the low intensity band in the subchondral zone of the femoral head (band sign) – a feature that is characteristic of osteonecrosis. Asymptomatic patient with primary antiphospholipid syndrome, from Khamashta 2000, with kind permission from Springer.

7.10.1 Osteonecrosis, Avascular Necrosis or Aseptic Necrosis

The prevalence of symptomatic osteonecrosis is 2–3% in APS patients, but up to 20% of PAPS may have asymptomatic osteonecrosis. Several factors have been associated with this disorder (Table 7.21), although the pathogenic mechanisms still remain partially elucidated. The most predominant hypotheses are included in Table 7.22.

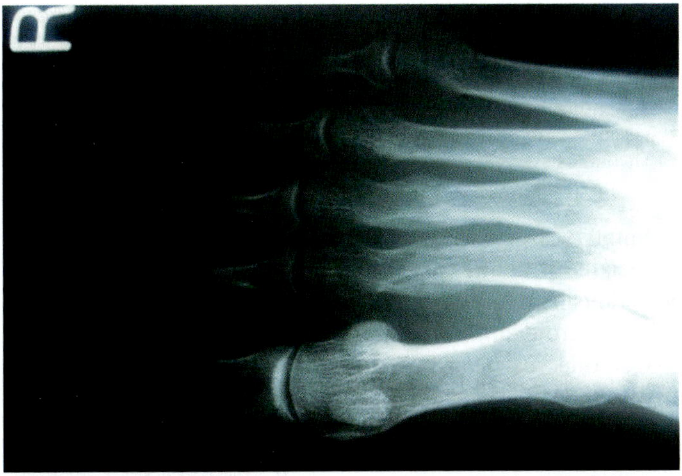

FIG. 7.19. Metatarsal fractures.

TABLE 7.21. Etiologic factors associated with osteonecrosis.

Trauma
Hematologic disorders: Sickle cell disease, Thalassemias, DIC, Polycythemia, Hemophilia, Clotting disorders.
Inherited thrombophilic factors: Protein C deficiency, Protein S deficiency, Antithrombin deficiency, Factor V Leiden, Homocysteinemia, Dysfibrinogenemia, decrease Tissue plasminogen activator, increase Plasminogen activator inhibitor.
Acquired thrombophilic factors: aPL, Nephrotic syndrome, Smoking, Alcohol, Pregnancy, Estrogens, Obesity, Diabetes mellitus, Cushing syndrome, Corticosteroids, Malignancies, Hepatic failure, Hyperlipidemia.
Connective tissue diseases (CTD): SLE, APS, RA, Systemic vasculitis, Systemic sclerosis.
Cytotoxic agents: vincristine, vinblastine, cisplatin, bleomycine, methotrexate, cyclophosphamide, 5-fluorouracil.
Infections: HIV, meningococcemia.
Metabolic conditions: Gaucher disease, Hyperparathyroidism, Hyperlipidemia, Hemodialysis, Renal transplant, Diabetes Mellitus, Gout.
Gastrointestinal diseases: Pancreatitis, Inflammatory bowel disease.
Others: radiation therapy, Legg-Calve-Perthes disease, dysbaric osteonecrosis, Fabry disease.

TABLE 7.22. Pathogenic mechanisms associated with osteonecrosis.

Mechanical vascular interruption (trauma, fractures)
Injury to or pressure on a vessel wall (vasculitis, infection, radiation, Gaucher disease)
Vascular embolism (fat, nitrogen bubbles, sickle cells)
Thrombosis

Small vessel vasulitis or thrombotic microvasculopathy associated with aPL have been suggested as the pathogenetic mechanisms in autoimmune diseases, even in the absence of corticosteroid administration.

Osteonecrosis can be entirely asymptomatic or it can be associated with pain and/or limitation of the movement in the affected joints. The most susceptible sites for osteonecrosis are the bones with single blood terminal supply such as the femoral head (the most vulnerable), the talus, the humerus head, or the carpal bones.

Early diagnosis is crucial in selecting the appropriate treatment options. Radiographic findings in early stages are unremarkable. In advanced disease, flattening, subchondral radiolucent lines (crescent sign), and collapse may be present. MRI is recognized as the most sensitive tool for the early recognition of osteonecrosis, having more than 95% overall sensitivity.

Treatment strategies primarily depend on the location, size and stage of the lesion. Conservative therapy, used in early stages, includes nonsteroidal agents or other analgesics for pain relief, steroid tapering, weightbearing avoidance, bed rest, or even immobilization for some cases. However, conservative therapies usually fail to prevent the progression of osteonecrosis. Thus, various prophylactic surgical procedures have been proposed in order to suppress the evolution of further degenerative changes (e.g., core decompression with or without bone grafting, osteotomy). Total joint arthroplasty is recommended for the late stage, which is characterized by necrotic subchondral bone, articular cartilage collapse, and secondary osteoarthrosis.

In patients with osteonecrosis and positive aPL, the use of anticoagulants might provide an effective therapy.

7.11 The Ear

The pathogenesis of sensorineural hearing loss (SNHL) is still considered idiopathic in most cases.

Evidence now exists that inner-ear pathology is frequently associated with immune dysfunction, including the presence of aCL in the sera of these patients. In fact, early corticosteroid and immunosupressor treatment has been associated with high improvement of symptoms.

Several autoimmune diseases have been associated with SNHL: SLE, Sjogren's syndrome, RA, ulcerous colitis, PAN, polymyositis, Hashimoto's thyroiditis, scleroderma, Behçet's disease, Cogan's syndrome.

Since the internal auditory artery is an end artery, disturbed circulation of the inner ear has long been suggested as the cause of sudden SNHL. Because microthrombosis associated with aPL is known to affect either dermal or retinal vasculature, a similar involvement of the cochlear vessels could be envisioned, causing sudden SNHL.

Sudden deafness, severe hearing loss of acute onset is usually unilateral, but may also occur bilaterally as well.

In addition to auditory symptoms, these patients may also present vestibular complaints, such as true vertigo, lightheadedness, or ataxia. Tinnitus and aural pressure are also frequent symptoms.

If suspected, the use of anticoagulant therapy in these patients may be considered.

7.12 The Eye

Ocular vaso-occlusive disease is a common finding in APS. aPL damage is predominant in the posterior segment as retinal or choroidal vaso-occlusive diseases and can be arterial, venous, or both. Visual aPL-related symptoms are shown in Table 7.23.

Anterior segment symptoms are less common, these include telangiectasias at conjunctival vessels, keratitis limbal or filamentary, and neovascular.

TABLE 7.23. aPL-related visual symptoms.

Decrease vision
Transient blurring
Amaurosix fugax
Transient diplopia
Field loss
Photopsy

Differential diagnosis should consider diabetic retinopathy, sarcoid, and hematological neoplasia, as well as stroke and accelerated artheriosclerosis, and of course systemic rheumatic diseases such as SLE, Sjögren's Syndorme or scleroderma, and some infections.

Prompt recognition and anticlotting therapy (aspirin and long-term oral anticoagulation) limit organ damage and usually achieve sustained improvement.

References

Amigo MC (2006) Kidney disease in antiphospholipid syndrome. Rheum Dis Clin North Am 32(3):509–522

Amigo MC, Garcia-Torres R, Robles M, Bochicchio T, Reyes PA (1992) Renal involvement in primary antiphospholipid syndrome. J Rheumatol 19(8):1181–1185

Asherson RA, Cervera R (2007) Pulmonary hypertension, antiphospholipid antibodies, and syndromes. Clin Rev Allergy Immunol 32(2):153–158

Asherson RA, Khamashta MA, Gil A, Vazquez JJ, Chan O, Baguley E, Hughes GR (1989a) Cerebrovascular disease and antiphospholipid antibodies in systemic lupus erythematosus, lupus-like disease, and the primary antiphospholipid syndrome. Am J Med 86(4):391–399

Asherson RA, Khamashta MA, Baguley E, Oakley CM, Rowell NR, Hughes GRV (1989b) Myocardial infarction and antiphospholipid antibodies in SLE and related disorders. Q J Med 73(272):1103–1115

Asherson RA, Higenbottam TW, Dinh Xuan AT, Khamashta MA, Hughes GRV (1990) Pulmonary hypertension in a lupus clinic: experience with twenty-four patients. J Rheumatol 17(10):1292–1298

Asherson RA, Cervera R, de Groot PG, Erkan D, Boffa MC, Piette JC et al (2003) Catastrophic antiphospholipid syndrome: international consensus statement on classification criteria and treatment guidelines. Lupus 12(7):530–534

Asherson RA, Frances C, Iaccarino L, Khamashta MA, Malacarne F, Piette JC et al (2006) The antiphospholipid antibody syndrome: diagnosis, skin manifestations and current therapy. Clin Exp Rheumatol 24(1 Suppl 40):S46–S51

Branch DW, Khamashta MA (2003) Antiphospholipid syndrome: obstetric diagnosis, management and controversies. Obstet Gynecol 101(6):1333–1344

Cabral AR, Cabiedes J, Alarcon-Segovia D (1990) Hemolytic anemia related to an IgM autoantibody to phosphatidylcholine that binds in vitro to stored and to bromelain-treated human erythrocytes. J Autoimmun 3(6):773–787

Castanon C, Amigo MC, Banales JL, Nava A, Reyes PA (1995) Ocular vaso-occlusive disease in primary antiphospholipid syndrome. Ophthalmology 102:256–262

Cervera R, Khamashta MA, Font J, Reyes PA, Vianna JL, Lopez-Soto A et al (1991) High prevalence of significant heart valve lesions in patients with the 'primary' antiphospholipid syndrome. Lupus 1(1):43–47

Cuadrado MJ, Mujic F, Munoz E, Khamashta MA, Hughes GRV (1997) Thrombocytopenia in the antiphospholipid syndrome. Ann Rheum Dis 56(3):194–196

Cuadrado MJ, Khamashta MA, Ballesteros A, Godfrey T, Simon MJ, Hughes GRV (2000) Can neurologic manifestations of Hughes (antiphospholipid) syndrome be distinguished from multiple sclerosis? Analysis of 27 patients and review of the literature. Medicine (Baltimore) 79(1):57–68

Derksen RH, Khamashta MA, Branch DW (2004) Management of the obstetric antiphospholipid syndrome. Arthritis Rheum 50(4):1028–1039

Espinosa G, Bucciarelli S, Cervera R, Lozano M, Reverter JC, de la Red G et al (2004) Thrombotic microangiopathic haemolytic anaemia and antiphospholipid antibodies. Ann Rheum Dis 63(6):730–736

Espinosa G, Bucciarelli S, Asherson RA, Cervera R (2008) Morbidity and mortality in the catastrophic antiphospholipid syndrome: pathophysiology, causes of death, and prognostic factors. Semin Thromb Hemost 34(3):290–294

Herranz MT, Rivier G, Khamashta MA, Blaser KU, Hughes GRV (1994) Association between antiphospholipid antibodies and epilepsy in patients with systemic lupus erythematosus. Arthritis Rheum 37(4):568–571

Hughes GR (2003) Migraine, memory loss, and "multiple sclerosis "Neurological features of the antiphospholipid (Hughes') syndrome. Postgrad Med J 79(928):81–83

Nesher G, Ilany J, Rosenmann D, Abraham AS (1997) Valvular dysfunction in antiphospholipid syndrome: prevalence, clinical features, and treatment. Semin Arthritis Rheum 27:27–35

Khamashta MA (2000) Hughes syndrome: antiphospholipid syndrome. Springer, London, p 474

Khamashta MA, Cervera R, Asherson RA, Font J, Gil A, Coltart DJ et al (1990) Association of antibodies against phospholipids with heart valve disease in systemic lupus erythematosus. Lancet 335(8705):1541–1544

McIntyre JA, Wagenknecht DR (2003) Antiphospholipid antibodies and renal transplantation: a risk assessment. Lupus 12(7):555–559

Meroni PL, Peyvandi F, Foco L, Bernardinelli L, Fetiveau R, Mannucci PM et al (2007) Anti-beta 2 glycoprotein I antibodies and the risk of myocardial infarction in young premenopausal women. J Thromb Haemost 5(12):2421–2428

Paran D, Chapman J, Korczyn AD, Elkayam O, Hilkevich O, Groozman GB et al (2006) Evoked potential studies in the antiphospholipid syndrome: differential diagnosis from multiple sclerosis. Ann Rheum Dis 65(4):525–528

Ruiz-Irastorza G, Khamashta MA (2007) Antiphospholipid syndrome in pregnancy. Rheum Dis Clin North Am 33(2):287–297

Sangle SR, D'Cruz DP, Jan W, Karim MY, Khamashta MA, Abbs IC et al (2003) Renal artery stenosis in the antiphospholipid (Hughes) syndrome and hypertension. Ann Rheum Dis 62(10):999–1002

Sangle S, D'Cruz DP, Khamashta MA, Hughes GR (2004) Antiphospholipid antibodies, systemic lupus erythematosus, and non-traumatic metatarsal fractures. Ann Rheum Dis 63(10):1241–1243

Sangle SR, D'Cruz DP, Abbs IC, Khamashta MA, Hughes GR (2005) Renal artery stenosis in hypertensive patients with antiphospholipid (Hughes) syndrome: outcome following anticoagulation. Rheumatology (Oxford) 44(3):372–377

Sanna G, Bertolaccini ML, Cuadrado MJ, Laing H, Khamashta MA, Mathieu A et al (2003) Neuropsychiatric manifestations in systemic lupus erythematosus: prevalence and association with antiphospholipid antibodies. J Rheumatol 30(5):985–992

Shoenfeld Y, Lev S, Blatt I, Blank M, Font J, von Landenberg P et al (2004) Features associated with epilepsy in the antiphospholipid syndrome. J Rheumatol 31(7):1344–1348

Stone S, Khamashta MA, Poston L (2001) Placentation, antiphospholipid syndrome and pregnancy outcome. Lupus 10(2):67–74

Stone S, Hunt BJ, Khamashta MA, Bewley SJ, Nelson-Piercy C (2005) Primary antiphospholipid syndrome in pregnancy: an analysis of outcome in a cohort of 33 women treated with a rigorous protocol. J Thromb Haemost 3(2):243–245

Suvajac G, Stojanovich L, Milenkovich S (2007) Ocular manifestations in antiphospholipid syndrome. Autoimmun Rev 6(6):409–414

Tektonidou MG, Malagari K, Vlachoyiannopoulos PG, Kelekis DA, Moutsopoulos HM (2003) Asymptomatic avascular necrosis in patients with primary antiphospholipid syndrome in the absence of corticosteroid use: a prospective study by magnetic resonance imaging. Arthritis Rheum 48(3):732–736

Tektonidou MG, Varsou N, Kotoulas G, Antoniou A, Moutsopoulos HM (2006) Cognitive deficits in patients with antiphospholipid syndrome: association with clinical, laboratory, and brain magnetic resonance imaging findings. Arch Intern Med 166(20):2278–2284

Toubi E, Ben-David J, Kessel A, Podoshin L, Golan TD (1997) Autoimmune aberration in sudden sensorineural hearing loss: association with anti-cardiolipin antibodies. Lupus 6:540–542

Uthman IW, Khamashta MA (2006) Livedo racemosa: a striking dermatological sign for the antiphospholipid syndrome. J Rheumatol 33(12):2379–2382

Uthman I, Godeau B, Taher A, Khamashta M (2008) The hematologic manifestations of the antiphospholipid syndrome. Blood Rev 22(4):187–194

Yehudai D, Shoenfeld Y, Toubi E (2006) The autoimmune characteristics of progressive or sudden sensorineural hearing loss. Autoimmunity 39(2):153–158

Chapter 8
aPL and Transplantation

Thromboembolic complications after transplant have been associated with inherited thrombophilic disorders, including deficiencies of antithrombin, protein C, protein S, factor V Leiden, the prothrombin G20210A and MTHFR C585C gene mutations, and dysfibrinogenemias.

Acquired disorders associated with transplant-related thrombosis include aPLs, malignancy, myeloproliferative disorders, heparin-induced thrombocytopenia, and hyperhomocysteinemia.

In the majority of the solid-organ and tissue transplants, the presence of aPL should be considered as a significant risk factor for any potential transplant candidate. So should it be in cases of prosthetic replacement surgeries.

The greatest risk is found in the first 6 months after transplantation. For some patients, however, the hypercoagulable state persists throughout life, and thrombotic loss of the transplanted organ can occur years after transplantation surgery. Peritoneal dialysis in patients awaiting renal transplantation appears to be at utmost risk.

Treatment for aPL-associated risks remains focused on intense anticoagulation therapy. Some patients, even on anticoagulant drugs, suffer aPL-related transplant failure. The use of immunosuppressive agents has not proven to have a marked effect on aPL titers, and has little effect on clinical events.

Given the serious psychological and economic impact of irreversible thrombosis in a transplanted organ, the modest

M.L. Bertolaccini et al., *Antiphospholipid Syndrome Handbook*,
DOI 10.1007/978-1-84628-735-0_8,

expense of pretransplant aPL screening should be readily justified. So should be in prosthetic replacement surgeries.

References

McIntyre JA, Wagenknecht DR (2003) Antiphospholipid antibodies and renal transplantation: a risk assessment. Lupus 12(7):555–559

Wagenknecht DR, Becker DG, LeFor WM, McIntyre JA (1999) Antiphospholipid antibodies are a risk factor for early renal allograft failure. Transplantation 68(2):241–246

Wagenknecht DR, Fastenau DR, Torry RJ, Becker DG, LeFor WM, Carter CB et al (2000) Risk of early renal allograft failure is increased for patients with antiphospholipid antibodies. Transpl Int 13(Suppl 1):S78–S81

Chapter 9
Differential Diagnosis

Any part of the venous circulation may undergo occlusion in APS. Deep and superficial veins of the lower limbs are most frequently involved, followed by PE and arm vessels. In these instances and in subjects who are relatively young (<45 years), the differential diagnosis rests on laboratory tests aiming at the identification of congenital or other acquired thrombophilic states (Table 9.1).

Some clinical features may point toward systemic disorders with a higher than average risk of venous thrombosis. For example, a history of oral and genital ulceration in a young person with venous thrombosis may suggest Behcet's disease, and the presence of peripheral blood eosinophilia could suggest the hypereosinophilic syndrome; conditions like APS do not spare any vascular bed.

When compared to the potentially recognized risk factors for venous thrombotic disease, there are fewer factors to consider in arterial thrombotic disease. All the other known risk factors for arterial thrombotic disease tend to produce thrombosis on the background of arteriosclerosis, so these patients tend to have recognizable risk factors for atherosclerosis, which should be controlled.

Special consideration should be given to stroke where up to 18% of young (<50) patients may have aPL. Some patients present with multiple cerebral lesions on magnetic resonance imaging. These types of lesions are also seen in multiple

M.L. Bertolaccini et al., *Antiphospholipid Syndrome Handbook*,
DOI 10.1007/978-1-84628-735-0_9,

Table 9.1. Differential diagnosis of venous thromboembolism in APS.

- Activated prot-C resistance/factor V Leiden (heterocygote and homozygous)
- Heterozygous deficiencies of:
o Antithrombin
o Prot-C
o Prot-S
- Prothrombin 20210 heterozygous or homozygous states
- Increased levels of factor VIII
- Myeloproliferative disorders and Malignancies (Trousseau's syndrome)
- Nephrotic syndrome
- Peripartum state
- Estrogen-containing oral contraceptives
- Behçet's syndrome
- Dysfibrinogenemia
- Heparin-induced thrombosis
- Hyperhomocysteinemia (possible risk factor)
- Paroxymal nocturnal hemoglobinuria (very rare)

Table 9.2. Multiple cerebral lesion in brain MRI: differential diagnosis.

- Multiple cerebral infarcts – microangiopathy
- Multiple sclerosis (MS)
- CADASIL (cerebral autosomal dominant arteriopathy with subcortical infarcts and leukoencephalopathy)
- Cerebral vasculitis

sclerosis (MS), in cerebral autosomal dominant arteriopathy with subcortical infarcts and leucoencephalopathy (CADASIL), and other conditions (Table 9.2).

CADASIL is a hereditary cause of stroke, migraine with aura, mood disturbances, and dementia. Thus if a patient does present with multiple cerebral lesions, a family history of stroke and dementia should be sought. The genetic defect has been mapped to chromosome 19 and can now be detected in the majority of major neuroscience centers.

On the other hand, it may be very difficult to differentiate APS from MS, since neurological manifestations and MRI can be indistinguishable. Both conditions can show oligoclonal bands in the CSF. Clues in those cases include a past history of venous thrombosis and pregnancy loss, suggesting APS, and the presence of atypical features of MS such as migraine or epilepsy, or other features such as livedo reticularis, sicca syndrome, Raynaud's, SLE features, or thrombocytopenia.

Evoked potential studies have been proposed as a useful tool to distinguish APS from MS, supported by the important differences described between both the groups. Abnormalities in these tests (especially in visual evoked potentials) are uncommon in APS patients, while they are quite common in MS patients.

Catastrophic APS has a number of clinical similarities to heparin-induced thrombocytopenia. In the latter, patients develop thrombosis at any site, both arterial, venous and microvascular (especially the skin). It usually develops within 10–14 days after starting heparin, and the first sign is a falling platelet count.

It should be differentiated from a transient thrombocytopenia that occurs in the first few days of heparin therapy, which is probably due to heparin causing platelet activation, and is not associated with any clinically harmful effects.

Hyperhomocysteinemia deserves a special mention for it is the only other condition related to pregnancy loss, arterial thrombosis, and possibly venous thrombosis. High plasma levels of homocystein result from the interplay between congenital and environmental factors (Table 9.3).

TABLE 9.3. Causes of hyperhomocysteinemia.

- Homozygous deficiency of cystathionine-β-synthase (the most common; prevalence of 1 in 3,35,000)
- Drugs (Methotrexate)
- Folate deficiency
- Homozygous state for the homocysteine MTHFR mutation C677T

aPL screen may also be indicated in other situations such as: thrombocytopenia, livedo reticularis, low levels of free prot-S (unknown mechanism), prot-C, and factor XII, and the presence of activated prot-C resistance.

Differential diagnosis of Pregnancy morbidity is discussed in another Chapter "Obstetric APS."

Chapter 10
Management of APS

10.1 Introduction

Long-term prognosis is most influenced by the risk of recurrent thrombosis in APS.

Therefore, the most important aspects concerning management of patients with APS are treating thrombosis, preventing re-thrombosis (i.e., secondary prophylaxis), and ideally, reducing the number of individuals having aPL who develop "the syndrome" (i.e., primary prophylaxis). A summary of the therapeutic recommendations is depicted in Table 10.1.

10.2 Primary Thromboprophilaxis in aPL-Positive Patients

Available data from clinical studies suggest that the thrombotic risk associated with aPL may be serious. In the general population, up to 5% of aPL positive patients will develop a thrombotic events; while in SLE patients, the risk for clotting complications is very high (50%).

Despite these data, the controversy concerning whether or not prophylactic treatment is indicated for patients with aPL who have no history of thrombosis remains unresolved.

M.L. Bertolaccini et al., *Antiphospholipid Syndrome Handbook*,
DOI 10.1007/978-1-84628-735-0_10,

TABLE 10.1 Management recommendations for APS.

1. *Antiphospholipid antibodies (aPLs) positive patient*: long term low dose aspirin (plus LMWH in high-risk situations)
2. *Antiphospholipid syndrome (APS) and thrombosis*:
   - (a) aPL positive + thrombosis
     - *Venous*: long term oral anticoagulation (INR 2.0–3.0)
     - *Arterial or severe venous thromboembolism*: long term oral anticoagulation (INR 3.0–4.0)
     - *Recurrent thrombosis (venous or arterial)*: long term oral anticoagulation (INR 3.0–4.0)
   - (b) *aPL positive + obstetric history (without previous thrombosis)*: long term low dose aspirin (plus LMWH in high-risk situations).
3. *Pregnancy morbidity*:
   - (a) *aPL positive without previous thrombotic history*: low dose aspirin . *Postpartum*: low dose aspirin + low dose LMWH (for 6 weeks)
   - (b) *aPL positive with previous obstetric history*:
     - *Early miscarriage (<10 weeks)*: low dose aspirin +/- low dose LMWH.
     - *Fetal loss (>10 weeks)*: low dose aspirin + low dose LMWH.
     - *All Postpartum*: low dose aspirin + low dose LMWH (for 6 weeks)
   - (c) *aPL positive with previous thrombotic history*: aspirin + high dose LMWH

Thus, low-dose aspirin (75 mg/day) is considered as a logical prophylaxis in individuals with persistently positive aPL and/or unequivocally positive LA tests; in case of aspirin allergy or intolerance, other antiaggregant drugs should be considered. Prothrombotic factors should be avoided (i.e., smoking, estrogen-containing oral contraceptive pills) and/or treated (i.e., hypertension, hypercholesterolemia, diabetes mellitus) in all patients. Furthermore, high-risk situations (such as surgery, long-haul travel) should be covered with subcutaneous heparin prophylaxis.

Hydroxychloroquine has well-documented antiplatelet effects and has been shown to reduce the risk of thrombosis in SLE patients.

10.3 Management of Thrombosis

Treatment of the acute thrombotic event, if identified, is not different in APS than in the general population.

There is now good evidence from both retrospective and prospective studies that APS patients with thrombosis will be subject to recurrences and that these can be prevented by long-term anticoagulation. Many patients with APS in whom anticoagulation has been stopped have had major recurrent thrombosis. Based on these data, indefinite oral anticoagulation has been accepted by most authors as the standard secondary prophylaxis for thrombosis in patients with APS.

It is not clear, however, whether prolonged anticoagulation is necessary in APS patients whose first thrombotic episode developed in association with surgery, oral contraceptive pill, pregnancy, or other circumstantial thrombotic risk factors.

The risk of recurrent thrombosis in patients with APS has been reported in between 22 and 69%. Usually, a venous thrombosis is followed by another venous thrombosis in more than 70% of cases. An arterial thrombosis is followed by another arterial thrombosis in more than 90% of cases.

Most patients requiring long-term anticoagulant therapy respond well to warfarin targeted to an INR of 2.0–3.0. However, intensity of anticoagulation should be individually targeted according to risk of thrombosis, thrombosis-related damage, and bleeding: patients with arterial events (specially stroke) and life-threatening pulmonary embolism should be maintained at INRs higher than 3.0; this target should be also indicated in patients who develop recurrent venous or arterial thrombotic events despite previous oral anticoagulation. A lower target INR could be acceptable for patients with non-severe venous thromboembolism.

The risk of intracranial and fatal bleeding in APS patients with previous thrombosis treated with oral anticoagulation to a target INR of 3.0–4.0 is low. Special caution must be paid to elderly patients, and patients with leukoaraiosis and/or previous serious bleeding.

Other risk factors for thrombosis such as smoking, hypercholesterolemia, hypertension, diabetes mellitus, and use of estrogens must be strictly corrected.

10.4 Management of Pregnancy Morbidity

Pregnant women with APS are at risk of complications at all stages of pregnancy. The early prediction of women who are likely to develop complications in pregnancy remains a challenge.

These patients require specialist care and a team approach involving obstetricians, obstetric physicians, internists, rheumatologists, hematologists, neonatologists, and specialist midwives. Close monitoring of the various aspects of the condition may reduce maternal morbidity and improve fetal outcome (Table 10.2). Under correct management, the likelihood of a live birth is between 85 and 90%.

Therapeutic options include aspirin, LMWH, and less commonly warfarin and steroids.

10.4.1 Aspirin

Women with APS are advised to take low-dose aspirin (75 mg/day) in pregnancy, and it is likely to be of more benefit if administered before conception. Treatment is usually continued beyond delivery.

Low-dose aspirin does not affect the use of regional anesthesia during labor. Renal and hepatic impairment do not occur with this dose of aspirin, and bronchospasm is exceptionally rare affecting a minority of asthmatics. There are no adverse fetal or neonatal effects from the use of low dose aspirin.

10.4.2 Heparin

Women with APS and a previous history of thromboembolism are treated with high dose of heparin (e.g., Enoxaparin 40 mg, SC, b.d.) as thromboprophylaxis in pregnancy (Table 10.3).

For those with recurrent pregnancy loss or previous adverse pregnancy outcome, but without a history of thromboembolism,

TABLE 10.2. Recommendations in APS pregnancy.

Recommendations
- *Preconceptional assessment.* Should include: detailed medical and obstetric history, documentation or confirmation of significant levels of aPL, review of medication, information of maternal and obstetric problems' risk and information of possible further treatments, blood tests (renal, blood cell count, liver, urine, ...). In those who have systemic lupus erythematosus (SLE), issues related to exacerbation of SLE also should be discussed. All patients should be assessed for evidence of anemia and thrombocytopenia, which occur in association with APS.
- *Detection of obstetric complications.* After week 20, close control of hypertension and proteinuria, and ultrasound examination every 4–6 weeks should be done. In the third trimester, "high risk" women with APS (e.g., abnormal Doppler assessment of the uterine arteries or previous late pregnancy complications) should be offered 2–4 weekly scans, whereas those at the milder end of the APS spectrum (e.g., recurrent first trimester losses only) may be offered scans at 28 and 34 weeks gestation. In cases with suspected fetal growth restriction, biophysical profiles should be performed to further assess fetal well-being.
- *Uterine artery Doppler*: Several studies have recommended uterine artery Doppler waveform analysis at 20 and 24 weeks gestation, since bilateral uterine artery notches at 22–24 weeks is associated with high likelihood for prediction of pre-eclampsia and fetal growth restricition (sensibility of 75%, specificity of 94%, negative predictive value of 94%).
- *Contraindications to pregnancy*: pulmonary hypertension, uncontrolled arterial hypertension, recent (<6 months) thrombotic event.

there is as yet no consensus of opinion. Some studies have demonstrated that heparin therapy in addition to aspirin may contribute to improve fetal outcome, especially in women with recurrent first trimester loss. In this case, low dose of LMWH (e.g., Enoxaparin 40 mg, SC, daily) is usually used as soon as pregnancy is confirmed. Although optimal treatment for women with one or more late pregnancy losses (second–third trimesters), but no history of thromboembolism is controversial, most obstetricians support the use of heparin therapy in addition to low-dose aspirin.

TABLE 10.3 Subcutaneous heparin regime used in the treatment of APS during pregnancy.

Recurrent pre-embryonic and embryonic loss; no history of thrombotic events
Unfractionated heparin(UFH):
1. 5,000–7,500 U b.d. in the first trimester
2. 5,000–10,000 U b.d. in the second and third trimesters
LMWH: Enoxaparin 40 mg or dalteparin 5,000 U o.d.
Prior fetal death or early delivery because of severe preeclampsia/ placental insufficiency; no history of thrombotic events
UFH:
1. 7,500–10,000 U b.d. in the first trimester
2. 10,000 U b.d. in the second and third trimesters
LMWH: Enoxaparin 40 mg or dalteparin 5,000 U o.d.
History of thrombotic events
UFH:
1. 7,500 U every 8–12 h adjusted to maintain the mid-interval heparin levels in the therapeutic range
LMWH: weight-adjusted (e.g., enoxaparin 1 mg/kg or dalteparin 200 U/kg b.d.)

The potential complications of heparin treatment during pregnancy includes hemorrhage, osteoporosis, fracture, and heparin-induced thrombocytopenia. The reported rate of osteoporosis and associated fracture is low, though cases have occurred. Whether LMWH during pregnancy is associated with decrease of bone density remains controversial. Calcium and vitamin D supplements may be added during this treatment. Heparin-induced thrombocytopenia is infrequent in pregnant women.

Although Factor Xa levels may be used to monitor LMWH, experience has shown that doses are virtually never altered as a result, and therefore it is not necessary to measure Factor Xa levels routinely.

Stopping LMWH administration at least 12 h prior to elective delivery or any interventional procedure, and reintroducing it 12 h after that is generally considered safe, but in case urgent delivery is necessary, reversal with protamine sulfate is possible.

The molecular weight of unfractionated heparin (UFH) ranges from 12–15 kD, and that of LMWH from 4–5 kD therefore neither preparation is able to cross the placenta. Heparin is not excreted into breast milk, and it is safe during breast feeding.

10.4.3 Warfarin

Warfarin is contraindicated in the first trimester because of its potential teratogenicity, particularly, on exposure of the fetus during weeks 6–12 of gestation. Switching to LMWH should be done either pre- or postconception, and usually it is maintained until postpartum. Heparin should be initiated at the time of warfarin cessation and should be continued until warfarin is reintroduced.

Warfarin may be needed in cases of recurrent thrombosis despite therapeutic doses of heparin. The INR must be controlled closely in these cases to minimize the probabilities of serious fetal bleeding.

There is no significant excretion of warfarin into breast milk.

10.4.4 Corticosteroids

The use of *corticosteroids* in APS pregnancies is rare except for the treatment of maternal thrombocytopenia or co-existent SLE, for which prednisolone is still first line therapy. Regular blood glucose monitoring is required with long-term administration of steroids. Patients requiring >7.5 mg prednisolone daily for more than 2 weeks prior to delivery should be given intrapartum intravenous hydrocortisone 100 mg tds. Breast feeding is rarely contraindicated, although women taking 60 mg prednisolone with healthy term babies may consider bottle-feeding because of the theoretical risk of neonatal hypothalamic-pituitary adrenal suppression at these high doses.

10.4.5 Other Drugs

Other drugs such as Azathioprine and Hydroxychloroquine can be safely used in pregnancy and breast feeding in cases of SLE-associated with APS.

10.5 Management of Thrombocytopenia

Thrombocytopenia in APS rarely requires treatment. When platelets are <50,000/mm^3, the treatment of choice are corticosteroids. Splenectomy could be performed in some patients with refractory thrombocytopenia. Anecdotal successful reports with other drugs (such as IVIG, Rituximab, Hydroxychloroquine, Aspirine, Dapsone, etc) have been published.

References

Branch DW, Khamashta MA (2003) Antiphospholipid syndrome: obstetric diagnosis, management and controversies. Obstet Gynecol. 101(6):1333–1344

Crowther MA, Ginsberg JS, Julian J, Denburg J, Hirsh J, Douketis J et al (2003) A comparison of two intensities of warfarin for the prevention of recurrent thrombosis in patients with the antiphospholipid antibody syndrome. N Engl J Med 349(12):1133–1138

Derksen RH, Khamashta MA, Branch DW (2004) Management of the obstetric antiphospholipid syndrome. Arthritis Rheum 50(4):1028–1039

Erkan D, Harrison MJ, Levy R, Peterson M, Petri M, Sammaritano L et al (2007) Aspirin for primary thrombosis prevention in the antiphospholipid syndrome: a randomized, double-blind, placebo-controlled trial in asymptomatic antiphospholipid antibody-positive individuals. Arthritis Rheum 56(7):2382–2391

Finazzi G, Marchioli R, Brancaccio V, Schinco P, Wisloff F, Musial J et al (2005) A randomized clinical trial of high-intensity warfarin vs. conventional antithrombotic therapy for the prevention of recurrent thrombosis in patients with the antiphospholipid syndrome (WAPS). J Thromb Haemost 3(5):848–853

Galindo M, Khamashta MA, Hughes GRV (1999) Splenectomy for refractory thrombocytopenia in the antiphospholipid syndrome. Rheumatology (Oxford). 38(9):848–853

Hunt BJ, Doughty HA, Majumdar G, Copplestone A, Kerslake S, Buchanan N et al (1997) Thromboprophylaxis with low molecular weight heparin (Fragmin) in high risk pregnancies. Thromb Haemost 77(1):39–43

Hunt BJ, Khamashta M, Lakasing L, Williams FM, Nelson Piercy C, Bewley S et al (1998) Thromboprophylaxis in antiphospholipid syndrome pregnancies with previous cerebral arterial thrombotic events: is warfarin preferable? Thromb Haemost 79(5):1060–1061

Hunt BJ, Gattens M, Khamashta M, Nelson-Piercy C, Almeida A (2003) Thromboprophylaxis with unmonitored intermediate-dose low molecular weight heparin in pregnancies with a previous arterial or venous thrombotic event. Blood Coagul Fibrinolysis 14(8):735–739

Khamashta MA (2000) Primary prevention of thrombosis in subjects with positive antiphospholipid antibodies. J Autoimmun 15:249–253

Khamashta MA, Cuadrado MJ, Mujic F, Taub NA, Hunt BJ, Hughes GRV (1995) The management of thrombosis in the antiphospholipid-antibody syndrome. N Engl J Med 332(15):993–997

Ostensen M, Khamashta M, Lockshin M, Parke A, Brucato A, Carp H et al (2006) Anti-inflammatory and immunosuppressive drugs and reproduction. Arthritis Res Ther 8(3):209

Ruiz-Irastorza G, Khamashta MA, Hunt BJ, Escudero A, Cuadrado MJ, Hughes GR (2002) Bleeding and recurrent thrombosis in definite antiphospholipid syndrome: analysis of a series of 66 patients treated with oral anticoagulation to a target international normalized ratio of 3.5. Arch Intern Med 162(10):1164–1169

Ruiz-Irastorza G, Hunt BJ, Khamashta MA (2007) A systematic review of secondary thromboprophylaxis in patients with antiphospholipid antibodies. Arthritis Rheum 57(58):1487–95

Appendix
Photographic Examples of Clinical Manifestations of APS

A.1 Skin Manifestations

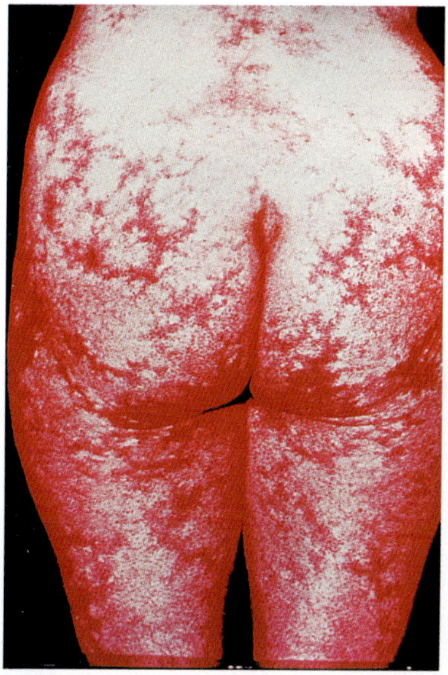

A.1.1. Livedo reticularis of the gluteal region and both thighs of a patient with SLE and APS, with kind permission from Springer-Verlag London.

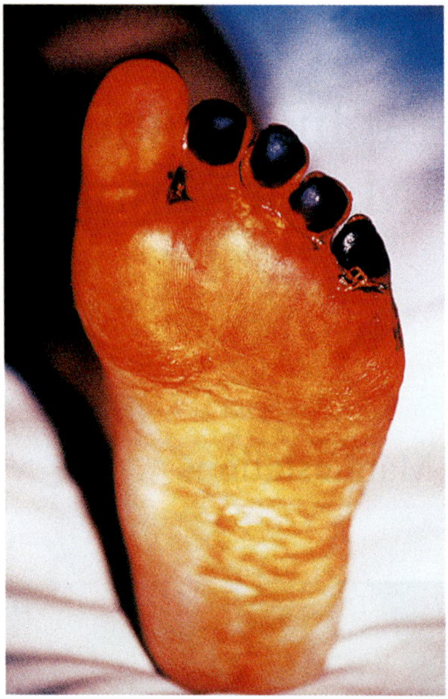

A.1.2. Evolution to gangrene with distal necrosis of the left foot toes in the patient carrier of primary APS, with kind permission from Springer-Verlag London.

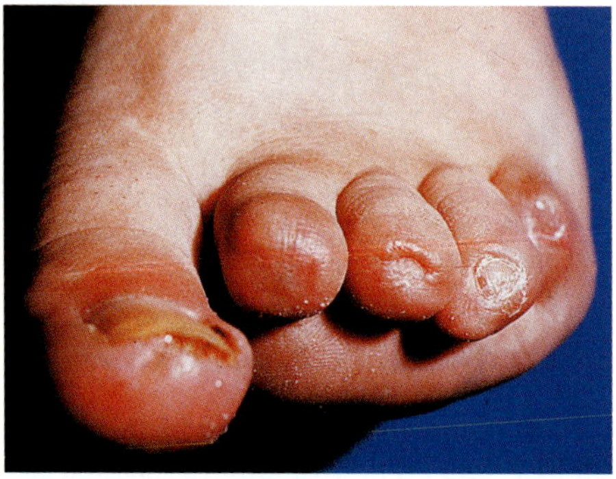

A.1.3. Cure by spontaneous amputation of the left foot toes affected with gangrene in a patient with primary APS, with kind permission from Springer-Verlag London.

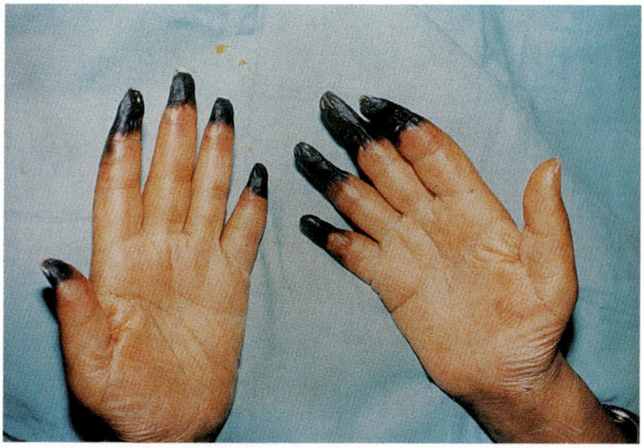

A.1.4. Digital necrosis with gangrene of the fingers of a patient with SLE and APS, with kind permission from Springer-Verlag London.

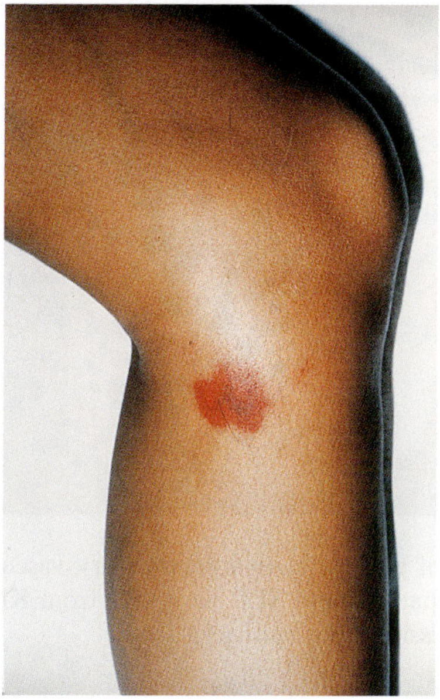

A.1.5. SLE along with APS presenting with papuloerythematosus skin lesion (irregular borders) on the lower limb, with kind permission from Springer-Verlag London.

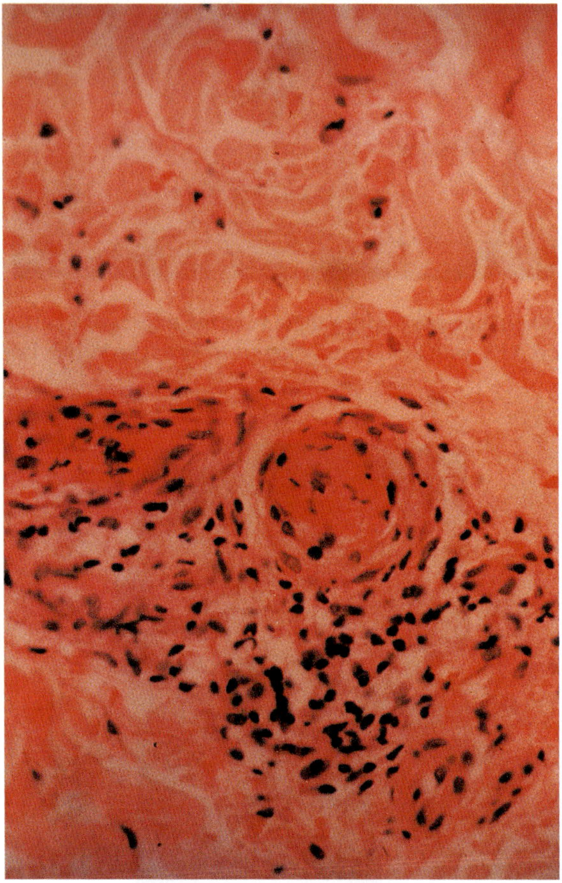

A.1.6. Biopsy of skin with noninflammatory vascular thrombosis (venular) of a patient with SLE and APS, from Khamashta 2000, with kind permission from Springer.

A.2 Renal Disease

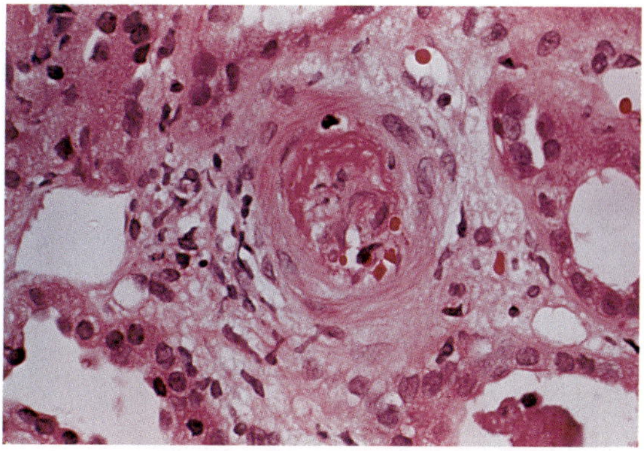

A.2.1. A small arteriole with a recent, almost occlusive, partially laminated thrombus. Some complete and fragmented white and red cells are seen (hematoxylin/eosin), with kind permission from Springer-Verlag London.

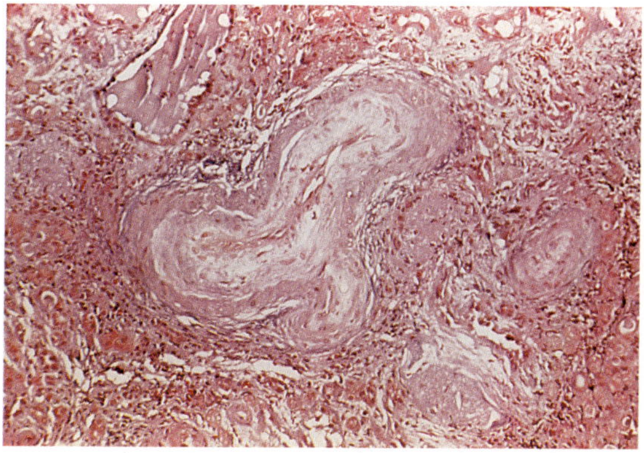

A.2.2. Typical histology of an interlobular arteriole which is almost occluded by a slightly cellular mucoid material. The lumen is distorted and the muscular media is partially destroyed and fibrotic. There is interstitial fibrosis with a moderate inflammatory infiltration. A dilated tubule containing hyaline material is seen (Masson), with kind permission from Springer-Verlag London.

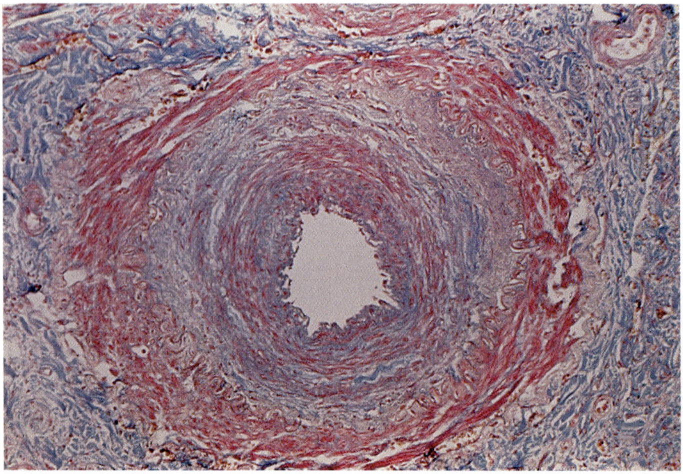

A.2.3. Chronic stage of an intraparenchymatous renal artery. Slight medial hyperplasia, fractures of the internal elastica, severe subendothelial fibrosis, myofibroblastic proliferation, and a drastic reduction of the lumen (Masson), with kind permission from Springer-Verlag London.

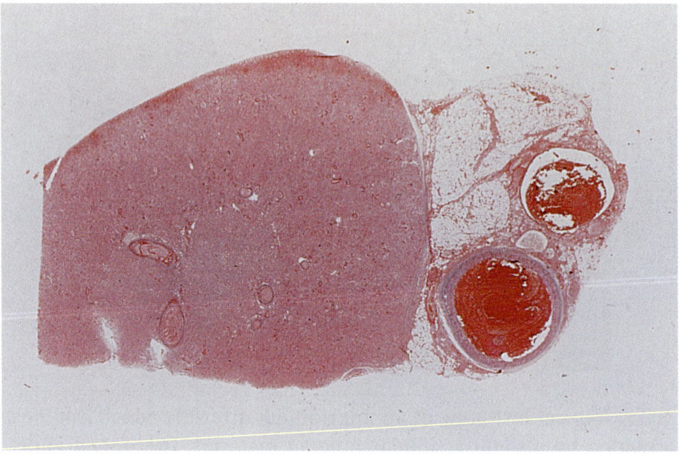

A.2.4. Fragment of the transplanted kidney in a female patient with PAPS. The whole vascular tree (from the intraparenchymatous vessels to the main intrarenal artery and vein) shows recent thrombotic occlusion (hematoxilin/eosin), with kind permission from Springer-Verlag London.

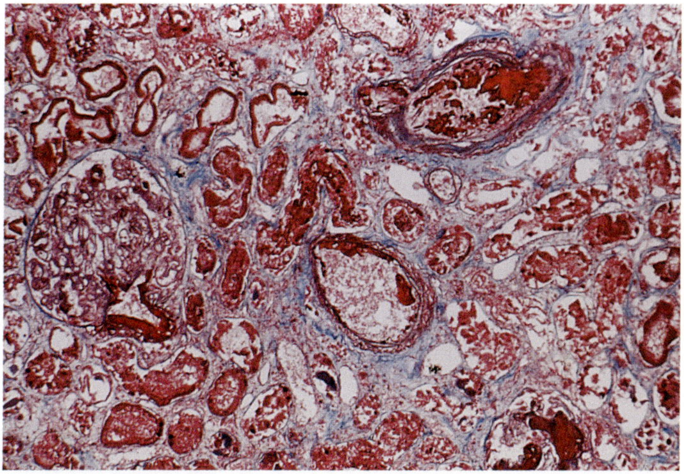

A.2.5. This micrograph belongs to the same kidney shown in Figure A.2.4. There is generalized thrombosis of the microvasculature including glomerular capillaries, afferent arterioles, and interlobular arteries. Generalized necrosis without inflammatory cell infiltration is also observed (Masson), with kind permission from Springer-Verlag London.

A.3 Obstetric Manifestations

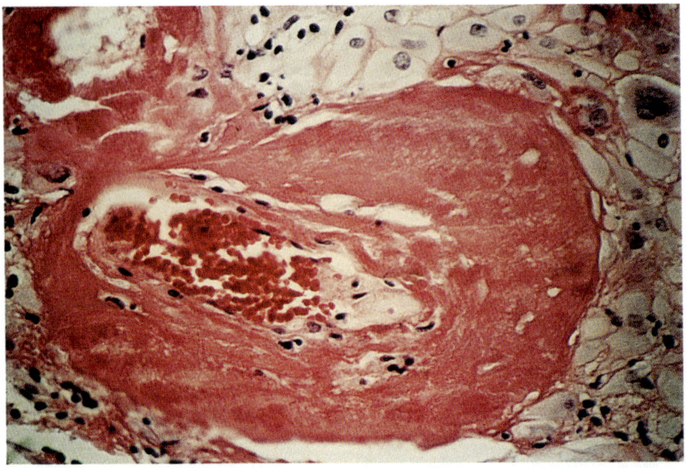

A.3.1. Decidual vessel showing fibrinoid necrosis, with kind permission from Springer-Verlag London.

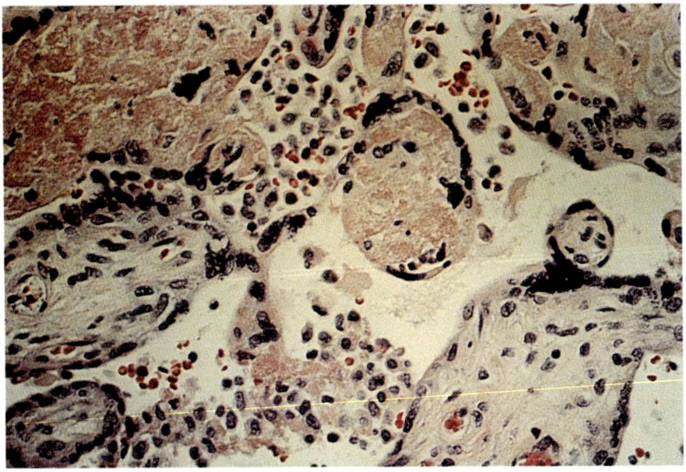

A.3.2. Placenta showing villitis and inter-villusitis, with kind permission from Springer-Verlag London.

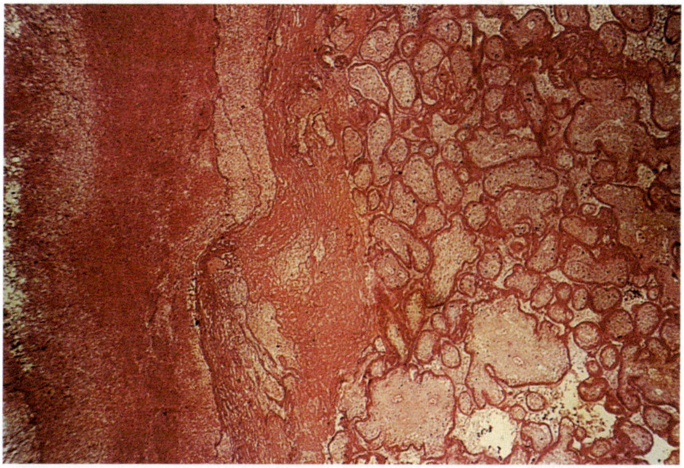

A.3.3. Thrombosed infracted villi in a patient with antiphospholipid syndrome, with kind permission from Springer-Verlag London.

A.4 Systemic Hypertension

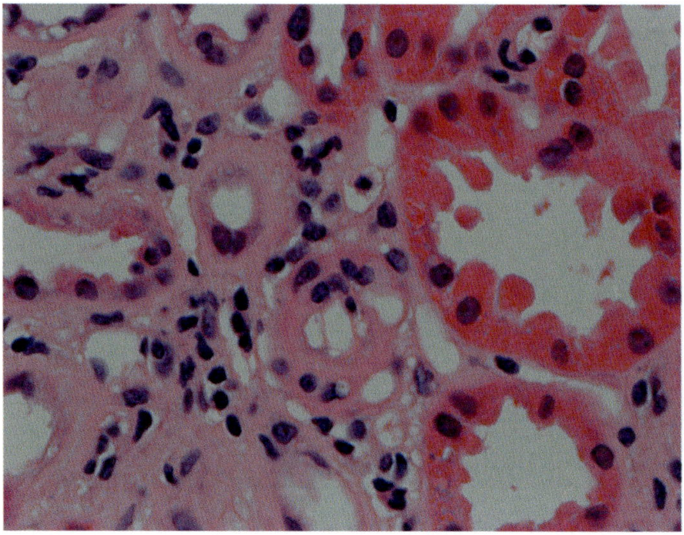

A.4.1. Renal thrombotic micro-angiopathy seen in a patient with APS and hypertension, with kind permission from Springer-Verlag London.

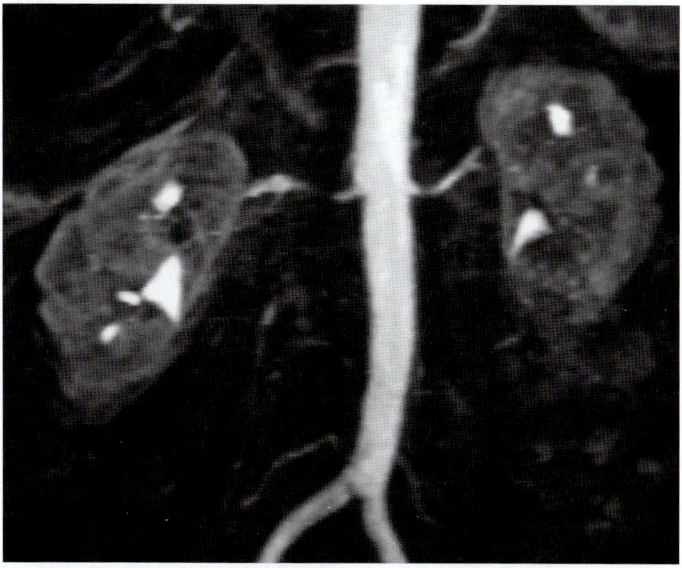

A.4.2. Magnetic resonance angiogram showing renal artery stenosis in a patient with APS and hypertension, with kind permission from Springer-Verlag London.

A.5 Osteoarticular Manifestations

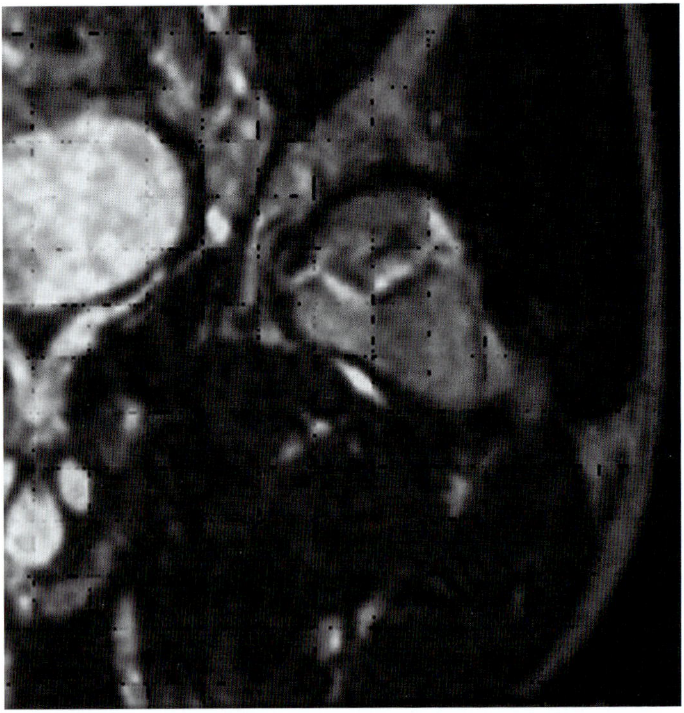

A.5.1. Osteonecrosis indicated by the presence of the double line sign (arrow) seen on T2-weighted spin echo image, with kind permission from Springer-Verlag London.

Index